T0296977

Historical origins of the concept of neurosis

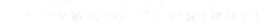

HISTORICAL ORIGINS OF THE CONCEPT OF NEUROSIS

JOSÉ M. LÓPEZ PIÑERO

Professor of the History of Medicine
University of Valencia

TRANSLATED BY D. BERRIOS

CAMBRIDGE UNIVERSITY PRESS
Cambridge
London   New York   New Rochelle
Melbourne   Sydney

CAMBRIDGE UNIVERSITY PRESS
Cambridge, New York, Melbourne, Madrid, Cape Town, Singapore, São Paulo, Delhi

Cambridge University Press
The Edinburgh Building, Cambridge CB2 8RU, UK

Published in the United States of America by Cambridge University Press, New York

www.cambridge.org
Information on this title: www.cambridge.org/9780521114714

© Cambridge University Press 1983

This publication is in copyright. Subject to statutory exception
and to the provisions of relevant collective licensing agreements,
no reproduction of any part may take place without the written
permission of Cambridge University Press.

First published 1983
This digitally printed version 2009

A catalogue record for this publication is available from the British Library

Library of Congress Catalogue Card Number: 82-19858

ISBN 978-0-521-24972-0 hardback
ISBN 978-0-521-11471-4 paperback

Contents

To Maria Luz

Introduction

Although the history of the concept of neurosis during the twentieth century can be said to be a direct continuation of the views of Charcot and Freud, it has created severe difficulties amongst historians; this problematic character partially results from the fact that it has been used as a battle ground by schools of thought such as the scientific-natural method, psychoanalysis and psychosomatic pathology. Over the years this has given rise to numerous attempts at reformulating the concept of neurosis, criticising its foundations and even eliminating it altogether.

Most authors agree on the usefulness of analysing the concept historically. In a meeting held in 1925, dedicated to a 'Revision of the Problem of the Neurosis', Oswald Bumke, a representative of the reaction of German academic psychiatry against psychoanalysis, stated:

> The first step in this revision is to obtain a clear view of
> what the term neurosis has meant in the past and means
> nowadays. As none of us would wish to resolve research
> questions by a majority vote, an attempt should be made to
> extract, from the historical evolution of the concept, ideas as
> to what direction the doctrine of neurosis might follow in
> the future.[1]

Unfortunately Bumke did not undertake nor encourage anyone else to do any historical research. He simply iterated few commonplaces about the evolution of the concept and used them to support his personal views. The same criticism can be levelled against most general studies on the neurosis and 'historical introductions' which are mostly based on second-hand information.

There is a clear difference between proper historical research and the simple outlining of an evolutionary map based on commonplaces, half truths and historical errors. This perfunctory style of historical writing, not uncommon amongst psychiatrists and physicians, reflects *inter alia* their attitude towards the historical disciplines. As Temkin[2] has lamented scientific standards are often not carried over from basic medical research to the historical field. Therefore, incomplete or misinterpreted data, which would suffice to disqualify a biochemical or genetic investigation, are often considered as acceptable in historical work.

Evolutionary accounts of the concept of neurosis limit themselves to enumerating 'landmarks'. The accustomed style is to start by producing a nebulous account of the work of Cullen and then follow this on with vignettes on Pinel and Charcot. The perfunctory treatment of these writers is then complemented by a detailed exposition of the Freudian views. No inquiry is ever made into the circumstances surrounding the emergence of the concept of neurosis and the pre-Cullean period is usually dispatched in a few glosses on the meanings of hysteria and hypochondria and on the manner these concepts were used in ancient medicine. The periods stretching from Cullen to Pinel and even from the latter to Charcot are passed over in silence.

Charcot's views on hysteria and on its psychogenetic origins started a new period in the history of neurosis and are at the very bases of current thinking on the subject. It would seem reasonable therefore to dedicate a monograph to the period of gestation (about which little is known) that preceded Charcot's work as it is during this time that the concept of neurosis took shape. This book, which is an abridged version of one of my earlier publications,[3] comprises four chapters, each corresponding to a specific stage in the evolution of the concept:

(1) The concept of neurosis was formulated for the first time in the same period that witnessed the development of medical science in its 'modern' sense; this reaction against traditional Galenism took place during the seventeenth and eighteenth centuries. The first chapter explores the manner in which such formulation shaped up under the new medical knowledge.

(2) The strong influence of *Naturphilosophie*, that romantic form of speculative medicine, placed German medicine in a pre-eminent position during the first half of the nineteenth century. The second chapter investigates how the concept of neurosis fared

under the impact of Naturphilosophie and of contemporary so-called 'eclectic' doctrines.

(3) The transformation in early nineteenth-century medical science and practice brought about by the Anatomoclinical School of Paris influenced the evolution of the concept of neurosis in a number of European countries. The third chapter describes the way in which this concept adapted itself to the new principle of anatomical lesion that characterized anatomoclinical medicine in the period prior to Charcot.

(4) During the middle of the nineteenth century the physiopathological and the anatomoclinical methods ran parallel. The fourth and final chapter examines changes in the concept of neurosis that resulted from the influence of the physiopathological view and outlines the emerging view of neurosis as a functional disturbance of the diseased organism.

This book intends to give an account of how the concept of neurosis was created and modified in response to the theoretical changes which occurred in medicine during two centuries. The historical epidemiology of the neurosis and cognate states is not touched upon and specific views on the concept of hysteria (and on other conditions falling under the neurosis umbrella) are mentioned only when relevant to the central question.

1: *The concept of neurosis*

The concept of 'neurosis' was coined by William Cullen, the Scottish physician, and appeared first in his *Synopsis Nosologiae Methodicae* (1769) and then in his *First Lines of the Practice of Physick* (1777).[4] In studies published between 1835 and 1841 three followers of the German Romanticism have disagreed with this fact and attributed the term to Felix Platter,[5] the Swiss physician of the Renaissance. This dissenting view, however, is based upon a misinterpretation of the term 'functionum laesiones', utilized by Platter in his treatise of practical medicine.[6] For Cullen the term 'neurosis' was no more than a useful neologism with which to refer to 'nervous disease', a concept current in the medicine of his time. Its meaning then, vastly different from the one in usage nowadays, embodies a view of neurosis that had currency before its anatomoclinical re-interpretation.

That the term 'nervous disease' had originated a century before was common knowledge amongst the writers who modified it during the second half of the eighteenth century and a number of studies available during Cullen's time echoed views from a British tradition that had been started by Willis and Sydenham. Cullen stated in *Synopsis*[7] (IV, p. 182) 'Since the time of Willis, British physicians have grouped some diseases under the category of nervous'. The Swiss Simon André Tissot, reported in his *Traité des Nerves et de leurs Maladies* (1778)[8] (written 10 years earlier): 'Sydenham... was the first to remark on the protean character of the nervous disease and to suggest that its symptoms might result from a disturbance in nervous function'. Additional evidence could be called upon to confirm the role played by Willis and Sydenham and to highlight the differences that came to separate the Galenic and modern views with respect to those diseases that 'we (eighteenth century writers) refer to as nervous'.[9]

1

The starting point: the views of Willis and Sydenham on 'Hysterical and hypochondriacal distempers'

Thomas Willis (1622–1675) was one of the main representatives of iatrochemistry during the second half of the seventeenth century. This movement, the first to formulate a medical system in the 'modern' sense, based itself upon the many ideas that had successfully challenged traditional Galenic medicine. In addition to the new chemical medicines and the Paracelsian view of disease, iatrochemistry included experimental and conceptual contributions as varied as the anatomical knowledge that had accrued from Vesalian reform; the doctrine of the circulation of the blood (and other physiological discoveries); the post-mortem search for anatomo-clinical correlations; the philosophical tenets of the inductive method and of the atomistic philosophy; and, the Cartesian view of man.[10]

Of the six books that constitute Willis's *Opera Omnia*, four are dedicated to the nervous system and its diseases. *Cerebri Anatome* (1664), one of the classical neuro-anatomical treatises of all times, suggests an iatrochemical re-interpretation of the traditional doctrine of the 'animal spirits'. The animal spirits are, according to Willis, made out of 'extremely subtle matter' and distilled from arterial blood in the cerebral cortex; therefrom animal spirits travel down the nerves to reach all regions of the organism where they are responsible for sensation and movement.[11]

In *Specimen* (1667) Willis included his views on 'cerebral and nervous pathology mainly in relation to epilepsy and other convulsive distempers'. In keeping with his iatrochemical views he used the term 'convulsive distempers' only in relation to diseases resulting from disorders of the nerves. Hysteria and hypochondria, which he considered as related but differentiable diseases, he included in this group. Hysteria 'the so-called uterine disease is primarily a convulsive disease caused by an alteration of the nerves and the brain'[12] and hypochondria is 'a spasmodic distemper' analogous to hysteria which involves the spleen and is also associated with a 'disorder of the animal spirits'.[13]

Willis wrote a book defending the 'nervous' or 'spasmodic' origin of hysteria and hypochondria against the view of Nathanael Highmore who had suggested as cause a haemodynamic alteration of the cardio-vascular system. Willis's work, *Affectionum quae*

The views of Willis and Sydenham 3

discuntur hysteriacae et hypochondriacae pathologia spasmodica vindicata (1670)[14] includes two important physiological sections.

De Anima Brutorum (1672), the fourth of Willis's neurological treatises, touches upon the notion of *'anima sensitiva'* and its pathogenic role. *'Anima sensitiva'* originates from the 'flamy and subtil' part of the blood and is responsible for aspects of animal life such as sensation, movement and impulse; its disorder may lead to cephalalgia, lethargy, somnolence, insomnia, vertigo, apoplexy, paralysis, delirium, melancholia, mania etc.[15]

Thomas Sydenham (1624–1689) made clinical observation the cornerstone of modern nosology. His empiricist stance led him to oppose all medical systems, particularly traditional Galenism and iatrochemistry, which had not yet freed itself from speculation. He sought to develop a new medical science which offered 'a graphic and natural description of disease' and was based on: (1) A classification into species of all clinical cases 'as carefully as it is done in botany'; in keeping with this desideratum Sydenham described the *morbid type* that is, a recurrent and typical way of becoming ill which can be identified by observing the regular patterns attending pathological phenomena; (2) A suspension of all theoretical preconceptions during the examination of the patient; and (3) A clear distinction, within each morbid type, between primary and accidental symptoms, the latter being associated with patient's variables such as age or response to treatment.[16]

Sydenham fulfilled his programme partially. He offered descriptions of morbid types such as hysteria to which he dedicated part of his *Dissertatio epistolaris* (1682), addressed to William Cole.[17] On the frequency of the condition Sydenham wrote: 'Of all chronic diseases hysteria...is the commonest; since just as fevers – taken with their accompaniments – equal two thirds of the number of all chronic diseases taken together, so do hysterical complaints (or complaints so called) make one half of the remaining third'[18] (T.N.: in English in the original). He emphasized the protean nature of hysteria, noticing that it may affect females (hysteria *sensu strictu*) and males (hypochondria) and suggesting as a possible cause 'ataxia or faulty disposition of the animal spirits'[19] (T.N.: in English in the original); i.e. he considered these conditions to be disorders of nervous function.

The view that hysteria and hypochondria resulted from a

disturbance of the nerves was a new one at that time and was put forward as an alternative to the Galenic doctrine that considered hysteria as caused by vapours that emanated from corrupt humours in the womb and hypochondria as resulting from vapours originating from 'atrabilis'; this term, that originally had meant 'black bile' or 'melancholia', was later used to refer to corrupt blood stagnating in organs placed in the hypochondria such as spleen, liver and stomach.[20]

The Galenic view had already come under attack in a book published in 1618 by Charles Lepois (Carolus Piso, 1563–1633) who claimed that hysteria could affect both sexes and, like epilepsy, resulted from accumulation of serum in the brain;[21] this modern view, however, is lost amidst traditional remarks. Although historically less influential, Lepois's contribution must be considered as an important antecedent to the work of Willis and Sydenham, the real originators of the concept of 'Nervous Disease'.

The emergence of the concept of 'nervous disease' marks the beginning of the 'modern view' both in neurosciences (Willis) and in nosology (Sydenham). Its 'modern' character emanates from the two basic postulates of the new medicine: firstly, that a unitary principle regulates all organic functions; and secondly, that nosology must be inductive in character and hence be based on clinical observation. This theoretical and experimental search for the unitary principle distinguishes modern from Galenic medicine and is founded upon the conceptual separation between form and function (made possible by Vesalius) which, in due course, led to the creation of two independent disciplines.

Renaissance medicine had already attempted (e.g. Giovanni Argenterio and Francisco Valles)[22] to identify a unitary principle by postulating that all traditional principles were under a superior regulator. When modern 'physiology' became an autonomous discipline during the seventeenth century, this regulator was identified with the nervous system. The 'nervous diseases' (what Cullen called 'neuroses') were believed to result from dysfunction in the unitary regulator. The novel feature of this concept (when compared to the traditional Galenic view) resides in the fact that it makes possible the identification of a group of conditions which can be considered both as functional and general in nature. As will be shown later, these two characteristics were to remain associated with the concept of neurosis for a long time to come. In a similar fashion, the inductive nosology developed by Sydenham allowed the concept of nervous disease to be clinically formulated in a way that had not been possible under the deductivist and essentialist control of the Galenic doctrine.

The consolidation of the concept of 'nervous disease'

During the first half of the eighteenth century the concept of 'nervous disease' became gradually clearer in spite of the fact that traditional views were still widely accepted.

Boerhaave, Hoffmann and Stahl, often called the 'great systematizers' for their contribution to the organization of medical knowledge, dealt with the concept of 'nervous disease' during the first ten years of the eighteenth century. Their views on hysteria and hypochondria can be considered as transitional between the old Galenic views and the new concept of 'nervous disease'.

Herman Boerhaave (1668–1738) synthesised, in an eclectic fashion, Cartesianism, iatromechanics (i.e. the application of Galilean mechanics to medicine), chemistry and the findings of post-mortem exploration. Following Sydenham, whose view he publicised, he considered clinical observation as the foundation of nosology. But classical views can also be detected in Boerhaave's work[23] as illustrated by the distinction between 'hypochondria *cum materia*' and 'hypochondria *sine materia*' in his *Aphorismi de cognoscendis et curandis morbis* (1709). Hypochondria *cum materia* he explained in terms of the old humoral doctrine of 'atrabilis'; hypochondria *sine materia* by means of the modern view of 'nervous mobility', that is of a 'proneness to action' in the 'animal spirits'.[24]

Also known as '*Communis Europae Praeceptor*', Boerhaave inspired many of his Dutch followers to adopt the twofold view of hypochondria. For example Gerhard van Swieten (1700–1772) founder of the 'alte Wiener Schule' or First Viennese school, included it in his *Commentaria in Hermanni Boerhaave Aphorismos* (1742) which became one of the most popular medical texts in Europe during the second half of the eighteenth century.[25] Joannes Oosterdijk Schacht (1704–1755), Boerhaave's successor in the Leyden chair, also classified melancholia into 'hypochondriacal or atrabiliary' and 'nervous or *sine materia*' in his *Institutiones medicinae practicae* (1747). Johannes de Gorter (1689–1762). Professor at Hardervijk and later physician to Elisabeth of Russia wrote at length on the concept of 'nervous mobility' in his *Praxis* (1750).[26] Physicians from other countries also adopted Boerhaave's dichotomous view but only Anne Charles Lorry (1726–1783), a successful clinician in pre-revolutionary Paris, will be mentioned; in his two-volume '*De melancholia et de morbis melancholicis*' (1753–1757) he defined 'nervous melancholia' as a spasmodic condition with manifold manifestations such as hysteria in the female and hypochondria in the male and believed that 'humoural melancholia' resulted from the action of the 'atrabilis' upon the nerves.[27]

Friedrich Hoffmann (1660–1742) developed a system based on a medical version of rationalistic mechanicism which was more speculative than Boerhaave's; according to this view all diseases can be reduced to alterations in 'tone' of the 'fibres' forming the solid parts of the body.[28] Hoffmann's views on hysteria and hypochondria were based upon a *sui-generis* combination of modern and traditional concepts. In his *Dissertatio* (1707) he considered these two conditions to be convulsive states that resulted from disorders of the womb and gut respectively, and which spread throughout the body by means of the spinal cord.[29]

The nosological views of Georg Ernst Stahl (1660–1734) do not live up to the expectations that his adoption of an animistic system may create in the historian. According to his doctrine 'anima' constitutes the activity principle of all vital phenomena, both in health and disease.[30] In his *Theoria medica vera* (1708) Stahl suggested that hysteria and hypochondria originated from a 'plethora' of blood in the portal vein which would obstruct the movement of 'animal spirits' and lead to alteration of the 'anima'.[31]

In addition to the contribution by the 'great systematizers', works on hysteria, hypochondria and the 'vapours' were published by other authors during the early eighteenth century. Traditional in conception, these writings followed either Galenic humoral views or iatrochemistry; amongst the latter should be mentioned the work of the British physicians John Purcell (1702) and Bernard de Mandeville (1711) who suggested that the conditions in question originated from 'imperfect digestion' or disorders in 'chyle formation'.[32] The terms hysteria and hypochondria are still utilized by these authors in their strict literal meaning, that is as referring to the role played by the womb, the hypochondria and the 'vapours'. Other works published during the same period sponsored a nervous pathology for the two conditions; amongst these a tendency can be detected to utilize hysteria and hypochondria synonymously with nervous disease. This explains why subsequent authors made free use of these two terms without feeling committed to a localizationalist hypothesis. By the same token eighteenth century physicians were able to retain the term 'vapours' in spite of the fact that they had already abandoned its especulative Galenic foundations. For example the French physician Dumoulin referred to vapours in his book of 1703 (which includes a free translation of Sydenham's work on hysteria), but rejected the claim that they reached the head from the lower abdomen, based on the observation that 'the organs in between are too solid and the blood vessels too full'.[33] Humphrey Ridley, a British neuro-anatomist of equal standing to Willis, also remarked upon the nervous origin of hysteria and hypochondria and provided a curious justification for referring to them as 'vapours', namely, that their cause can be dissipated easily in comparison with the aetiology of other affections.[34] Pierre Pomme in his *Traité des affections vapoureuses des deux sexes* (1765) published only two years before Cullen's work, also employed the term 'vapours' but with a meaning unrelated to the old doctrine of humours: '"vapourous disorders" refer to diseases of nervous origin whether general or particular, that give rise to irritability and spasm. In women these are called hysterical and in men hypochondriacal'.[35]

The concept of nervous disease became consolidated in a number of monographs published by British authors during the middle of the eighteenth century. In chronological order these are: Richard Blackmore's *A Treatise of the Spleen and Vapours; or Hypochondriacal and Hysterical Affections* (1728) and Nicholas Robinson's *A New System of the Spleen, Vapours and Hypochondriacal Melancholy* (1729). George Cheyne's *The English Malady: or a Treatise of Nervous Diseases of all Kinds, as Spleen, Vapours, Lowness of Spirits, Hypochondriacal and Hysterical Distempers* appeared in 1733 and Malcolm Flemyng's *Neuropathia: sive de morbis hypochondriacis et hystericis*, written in verse,[36] was published in 1740. After the publications of some minor monographs, such as Charles Perry's[37] *A mechanical account and explication of the Hysteric Passion* (1755), this series culminated with *Observations on the nature, causes and cure of those Disorders which are commonly called Nervous, Hypochondriac or Hysteric* (1765)[38] by Robert Whytt, who preceded Cullen in the Edinburgh chair. The French translation of Whytt's important book (1767) published two years before Cullen utilized the term 'neurosis' for the first time, contained a translator's appendix entitled 'Summary of the main works on the nature and causes of nervous, hysterical and hypochondriacal disorders' which mentioned about thirty-five works. This addendum illustrates well, in spite of the uneven quality of the listed contributions, the level of conceptual organization reached by the notion of 'nervous disorder' and shows that at the time there was already awareness of its novelty in relation to more traditional doctrines.[39]

The above-mentioned monographs have as common denominator the view that a class of diseases can be identified which have 'nervous' origin; beyond this individual authors differed markedly as they described the putative mechanisms in terms of their own theoretical systems. For example Blackmore continued referring to changes in 'animal spirits'; Robinson, Flemyng and Perry resorted to iatromechanical hypotheses; Cheyne propounded an eclectic integration of iatrochemistry, iatromechanics and Stahlian views; Whytt supported the doctrine of 'sympathy'.

It would not be wrong to say that the various terms included in the titles of the monographs represent each the conceptual vestige of an old pathogenic theory and in the case of terms such as 'vapours' or 'spleen' their origin is not difficult to identify. The development of new theories rendered some of these terms unsuitable or obsolete (as is the case with hysteria in the present century) and more adequate replacements were required. This historical mechanism might explain the popularity achieved by the term 'nervous disease', included by both Cheyne and Whytt in the title of their books. The same concept was occasionally referred to by means of neologisms; one such was 'neuropathia', coined by Flemyng twenty-five years before Cullen's main publication. In countries, such as France, however, the term 'vapours' was maintained for example in the work of Raulin and Pomme; this was also the case with Whytt's book which was translated as *Les vapeurs et les maladies nerveuses, hypochondriaques et hystériques.*[40]

British authors called some of these 'nervous distempers' 'English', probably on account of an assumed high local prevalence. Thus when writing on 'English spleen' Blackmore stated:

> If a phthisis is justly called by foreigners *Tabes Anglica*, or the English consumption, because it is most predominant, and in a manner peculiar to this country; I am well assured there is no less reason to give to the distemper I have chosen for the subject of this treatise, the appellation of the English spleen; since it is here gained such a universal and tyrannical dominion over both sexes, as incomparably exceeds its power in other nations[41]

(T.N.: in English in the original). In his *English Malady* Cheyne wrote: 'These nervous disorders being computed to make almost one third of the complaints of the people of condition in England'.[42]

The series of monographs mentioned above culminated with the publication of a book by Robert Whytt (1714–1766). This important figure of the European Enlightenment trained in Edinburgh, London and later in Paris and Leyden, and became Professor of Medicine at Edinburgh in 1746. With Haller he crossed swords on the topic of irritability and sensibility, was accused of following Stahl but soon disowned by the Stahlians. Whytt's experimental work is impressive: he showed that the spinal cord is necessary to reflex function; described the pupillary light reflex and demonstrated that it is interrupted by damage to the anterior quadrigemina; he also contributed to the clinical description of 'dropsy of the brain' or hydrocephalus.[43]

In his *Observations* (1765) Whytt wrote:

> the disorders which are the subject of the following observations have been treated of by authors, under the name of flatulent, spasmodic, hypochondriac or hysteric. Of late, they have also got the name of *nervous*, which appellation having been commonly given to many symptoms seemingly different, and very obscure in their nature, has often made it be said that physicians have bestowed the character of *nervous* on all those disorders whose nature and

causes they were ignorant of. To wipe off this reproach, and, at the same time to throw some light on nervous, hypochondriac and hysteric complaints, is the design of the following observations.[44]

(T.N.: in English in the original).

Whytt's view is that 'nervous diseases' result from a pathological alteration of the mechanism of 'sympathy'. 'Sympathy' refers to the type of relationship that organs hold with one another and describes a type of sensibility conveyed by the nerves:

All diseases may, in some sense, be called affections of the nervous system, because, in almost every disease, the nerves are more or less hurt; and, in consequence of this, various sensations, motions, and changes, are produced in the body. However, those disorders may, peculiarly, deserve the name of *nervous*, which, on account of an unusual delicacy, or unnatural states of the nerves, are produced by causes, which, in people of a sound constitution, would either have no such effects, or at least in a much less degree[45]

(T.N.: in English in the original).

'Nervous disease' became a fashionable diagnosis because of Whytt's reputation. James Makittrick Adair in his *Medical Cautions* (1786) bore witness to this twenty years later:

Upward of thirty years ago, a treatise on nervous diseases was published by my quondam learned and ingenious preceptor, Dr. Whytt, Professor of Physick, at Edinburgh. Before the publication of this book people of fashion had not the least idea that they had nerves; but a fashionable apothecary of my acquaintance, having cast his eyes over the book, and having been often puzzled by the enquiries of his patients concerning the nature and causes of their complaints, derived from thence a hint, by which he readily cut the gordian knot – '*Madam, you are nervous*'; the solution was quite satisfactory, the term became fashionable, and spleen, vapours and hyp were forgotten[46]

(T.N.: in English in the original).

The influence of Whytt was felt not only locally or by those belonging to social classes which were 'à la mode', it rapidly spread to continental physicians as is attested by the French translation of Whytt's *Observations* in 1767.

There was general agreement amongst authors that the core conditions of the class 'nervous disease', were hysteria and hypochondria, in the sense they had been defined by Sydenham; some followed his unitary view; others preferred a dichotomic approach. In addition to hysteria and hypochondria, later called 'major neuroses', there was a third distemper called by Whytt 'simple nervous disorder': subjects suffering from this, he stated 'though usually in good health, are yet, on account of an uncommon delicacy of their nervous system, apt to be often affected with violent tremors, palpitations, faintings and convulsive fits, from fear, grief, surprise, or other passions; and from whatever greatly irritates or disagreeably affects any of the more sensible parts of the body'[47] (T.N.: in English in the original).

The term 'nervous disease' meant for writers before Cullen (who only applied it to hysteria and germane conditions) something different from the 'neurological' meaning it has in the present time. This meaning developed fully only during the first half of the nineteenth century after the work of Abercrombie, Ollivier d'Angers, Romberg and the other founders of neurology.[48] Glimpses of this meaning however can be caught in Tissot's *Traité des neurfs et de leurs maladies*,[49] in Boerhaave's[50] lectures on 'de morbis nervorum' (1761) and even in Willis's work. In Cullen's writing the two meanings of 'nervous disorder' are still inextricably combined and only became separated during the anatomoclinical period. This blending of meanings in Cullen's work was to have important consequences for the evolution of the concept of neurosis.

The concept of neurosis in Cullen

William Cullen (1710–1790) was one of the great physicians of the Edinburgh school during the last third of the eighteenth century. After penurious college years he obtained his doctorate in medicine from Glasgow University where he became Professor in 1751. In 1755 he was appointed Professor of Chemistry at Edinburgh, in 1766 he acceded to the chair of 'Institutes of Medicine' and in 1773 to that of the 'Practice of Physic' in the same University. His work, known through translations in most continental countries, became extremely influential. He was nonetheless no creator, his mind and style being those of a lucid compiler. Still he was able to anchor whatever medical knowledge there was in his time upon the secure foundation of clinical practice.[51]

Although trained on the principles of Boerhaave's system Cullen later rejected the explanations of disease propounded by the Dutch physician. He expressed far less admiration for Hoffmann, but was strongly influenced by his views on solidism and on the role played by the nervous system in the maintenance of 'tone' in the organic fibre. He showed little interest in Stahl's views which he considered to be speculative.[52]

Cullen's system can be considered as a version of vitalism, a doctrine developed during the Enlightenment as an offshoot of the hallerian concept of 'irritability'. He was the best representative of the school of so-called 'neuropathology' (or neuralpathology) whose main postulate was the identification of the vital principle with the activity of the nervous system.

The nervous system had already acquired great importance in the work of Haller. Vitalist writers, even those not interested in 'neuralpathology', gave a great deal of attention to the nervous system, which stimulated progress in its anatomy, physiology and pathology. For example, during the period immediately prior to Cullen, the followers of Stahl emphasized the role played by the nervous system as the instrument of the 'anima'; likewise the Hoffmannians were led to the nervous system by their interest in the concept of 'tone'. These early associations and shifts in the direction of research paved the way for future growth.

The development of conceptual links between 'vis nervosa' and 'irritability' led to a form of vitalism which considered the nervous system as the physiological foundation of the body and of life itself; all diseases therefore could be reduced to being 'nervous alterations'. Cullen was not the sole originator of this doctrine and parallel 'neuralpathology' systems[53] were developed by Albrecht Thaer in Germany and David MacBride and Jacob Mackintrick in Great Britain.

'Tone' and 'irritability' in the solid part constitute the primary manifestations of life. 'Tone' for Cullen was not, as it had been for Hoffmann, an inherent characteristic in tissues but a property transmitted to it by the nervous system. The fluid that transmitted this property was conceived of by Cullen as similar to 'ether', thus showing the influence of Newton on eighteenth century British

Medicine. Reduced availability of the fluid would lead to 'atonia' and excess to 'spasm'; the two resulting polar categories constituting the basic pathological states.

Cullen subscribed to *more botanico* taxonomy. Before him, however, a number of classifications had appeared inspired by Sydenham's injunction that diseases should be organized in 'discreet and well defined species, in the way done by botanists'. During the second half of the eighteenth century this taxonomic approach led to ontological interpretations and diseases were considered as natural kinds susceptible to classification into classes, families, genera and species. Sauvages, a Professor at Montpellier, published in 1760 one of the earliest classifications of this kind; he was soon followed by the botanist and physician Linné (1763) and by Vogel (1764) a Professor at Göttingen. Cullen's *Synopsis Nosologiae methodicae*, where the term 'Neurosis' was mentioned for the first time,[54] appeared five years later.

Cullen's concept of neurosis finds its roots in 'neuralpathology' and in *more botanico* taxonomy. In his *First lines of the Practice of Physick* (1777) he stated: 'In a certain view, almost the whole of the diseases of the human body might be called nervous, but there would be no use for such a general appellation; and, on the other hand, it seems improper to limit the term in the loose inaccurate manner in which it has hitherto applied, to hysteric and hypochondriacal disorders, which are themselves hardly to be defined with sufficient precision'[55] (T.N.: in English in the original). This paragraph criticizes Whytt's concept of 'nervous disease' and introduces a view obtained by Cullen from 'neuralpathology', namely that the term 'nervous' should be used to refer only to diseases originating from direct alterations of the nervous system and not to diseases only indirectly considered as 'neurogenic'. But he also disagreed with restricting the use of the term to hysteria and hypochondria as had been done by Whytt and followers. He chose a *via media* according to which all 'nervous diseases' ('neuroses') were grouped into a discrete *class* in his classification, a class however with a wider membership than the Whyttian 'nervous disorder'.

Cullen separated in his classification general from local diseases. General diseases comprise the first three classes, namely: I 'Pyrexiae'; II 'Neuroses'; and III 'Caquexiae'; local diseases consist of only one class, IV 'Locales'. In the *Synopsis*, neuroses are defined aphoristically as 'Sensus et motus laesi sine pyrexia et sine morbi locali'.[56] In the *First Lines of the Practice of Physick* he amplified this view:

> In this place I propose to comprehend, under the title *neuroses*, all those preternatural affections of sense and motion, which are without pyrexia as a part of the primary disease; and all those which do not depend upon a topical affection of the organs, but upon a more general affection of the nervous system and of those powers of the system upon which sense and motion more specially depend[57]

(T.N.: in English in the original). This definition, often misinterpreted, provides negative criteria to separate the neuroses from the other '*classes*' and at the same time emphasizes their direct dependence upon dysfunction of the nervous system. Its main criterion however cannot be considered to be an absence of anatomical lesion because the theoretical principle this embodied was not yet part of Cullen's conceptual system; it was only during the anatomoclinical period that the concept of anatomical lesion was erected as a defining criterion for all true morbid states. Although Cullen included into his class of neuroses morbid entities known to have an anatomical lesion, the proper use of the anatomopathological principle came only with Pinel twenty years later.

The *class* 'Neuroses' is subdivided by Cullen into four *orders*: I 'Comata'; II 'Adynamiae'; III 'Spasmi'; and IV 'Vesaniae'. In doing this his intention had been (as he admitted) to bring together under a new class conditions which in the systems of Sauvages, Linné and Vogel had been classified under four different classes. Indeed Linné had already adumbrated at a grouping of this kind when he referred to the *morbi nervini* as a possible category to subsume four of his *classes*. Cullen indicated the provenance of each of the conditions forming his new *class*:

I *Comata* reduced voluntary movements, with drowsiness or unconsciousness). It corresponds to: Sauvages CL. VI; Ord. II;[58] Linné, CL. VI: Ord. II (*Soporosi*); Vogel, CL. VI (*Adynamiae*).

II *Adynamiae* (diminished involuntary movements, whether vital or natural). It corresponds to: Sauvages, CL. VI; Ord. IV (*Leiopopsychiae*); Linné, CL. VI, Ord. I (*Defectui*); Vogel, CL. VI.

III *Spasmi* (abnormal movement of muscles or muscle fibres). It corresponds to: Sauvages, CL. IV.; Linné, CL. VII. (*Motorii*) Vogel, CL. V.

IV *Vesaniae* (altered judgement without coma or pyrexia) 'under this name I suggest a special *order* of diseases equivalent to Vogel's *class* IX which he names *paranoias*. It is however different from the *vesaniae* as defined by Sauvages and Sagar in that my category does not include any of the *orders* which these authors call hallucinations and morosities. Likewise it can be differentiated from Linné's class of *mentales* in that my category does not contain his *morbi imaginarii* and *pathetici*'.[59]

Like other taxonomic systems during that period Cullen's *orders* are subdivided into *genera* and these into *species*. The number of species brought into the category neurosis is large: 'Comata' comprise apoplexy and paralysis; 'Adynamiae' include syncope, dyspepsia, hypochondria and chlorosis; 'Spasmi' group tetanus, trismus, epilepsy, palpitations, asthma, whooping cough, pyrosis, cholic, diarrhoea, diabetes, hydrophobia and hysteria; and 'Vesaniae' include amentia, melancholia, mania and somnolence.

Cullen's work is important to the history of the neuroses in a number of ways. First of all he gave origin and currency to a term still in use nowadays, its diffusion was helped by Cullen's commanding reputation and by the multiple foreign versions of his books. Pinel also helped by introducing the term in France and giving it an anatomoclinical interpretation.

Cullen defined the neuroses as morbid states caused by pathological processes which were both physiological and general and insisted that the neuroses never resulted from local but from 'general alterations of the nervous system';[60] the latter he identified as the unitary regulator of all organic functions and as the principle of life. Cullen's clear-cut definition was to clash, in the fullness of time, with the anatomoclinical view and its central principle, namely that all diseases can be reduced to an anatomical lesion. The history of the concept during the nineteenth century shows the anatomoclinical view setting limits upon what conditions could legitimately be included under the class neurosis. This process of contraction continued unabated through decades until hysteria and germane states became the only morbid states left in the group. By then the wheel had turned full circle with the remaining neuroses being the very ones that had been classified as nervous disorders before Cullen broadened the concept.

The concept of neurosis from Cullen to the beginning of the anatomoclinical period

The concept of neurosis underwent no change during the immediate post-Cullean period: medicine continued as it had been in the writings of the Scottish author and Vitalism, under various guises, remained as the doctrinal underpinning of pathology and maintained its close links with *more botanico* taxonomy. This section deals with the diffusion of Cullen's view and with its interaction with contemporary rival doctrines.

Cullen's work held sway in British medicine during this period. His *Synopsis nosologiae* went through three editions (two in Latin and one in English) and in abridged form was included in a number of treatises on the classification of disease. The *First Lines of the Practice of Physick, Institutions of Medicine, Clinical Lectures* and *Lectures on the materia medica* also went through a number of English editions. His disciples adopted the term 'neurosis' to name a *class* of disease: for example, Andrew Duncan from the Edinburgh School did so in his nosological system (1778); likewise the American David Hosack, whose book of 1821 can be considered as the culmination of this type of work in English medical literature.[61]

A group of psychiatrists influenced by Cullen (Arnold, Prefect, Crichton, Pargeter) also adopted the term 'neurosis'; for example Crichton used the term descriptively in his book on mental diseases (1798).[62] Other authors, although trained at Edinburgh and in agreement with Cullen's general classification, preferred other terms; thus Thomas Young (1813) used *paraneurismi*, and the Austrian Frank X. Swediaur (1802) wrote on *dycrethesiae et dysaesthesiae*.[63]

Other works from this period also deserve mention. Three years after Cullen's *Synopsis*, David MacBride (1726–1776) published his nosological system which was based on 'neuralpathology' and contained summaries of the classificatory schemes of Sauvages, Linné, Vogel and Cullen and also of the work by Johannes B. Sagar[64] which appeared in 1771. MacBride included four *classes*: (1) Universal diseases; (2) local or topical diseases; (3) sexual diseases; and (4) childhood diseases.

Universal diseases are 'those which may occur at any age, affect either sex and are characterized by a predominance of general over local symptoms'.[65] Amongst the fifteen general symptoms that are supposed to characterize them MacBride included excessive heat, cold, nausea, thirst, pain, pruritus, insomnia, somnolence, anxiety, laboured breathing, weakness, spasm, anaesthesia, hyperaesthesia and delirium.

'Universal Diseases' are subdivided into eight *orders*. The first three, 'fever', 'inflammation' and 'flux' depend upon 'excessive and abnormal motility of the vascular system combined with a disorder of the nervous system'.[66] The next three *orders* 'pain', 'spasm' and 'weakness' 'relate to the nervous system and are believed to originate from heightened, lowered or intermittent movements in its solid parts'[67] and form a group which MacBride could have named 'neurosis' or 'nervous diseases'. He grouped 'pain', 'spasm' and 'weakness' in terms of a neuralpathological criterion similar to Cullen's, namely their 'purely nervous'[68] nature which contrasted with the 'partial' nervous quality of the first three *orders*. MacBride never coined a term to name this group but kept it separate; his reference to Hoffmann and Whytt[69] in this context is significant.

One of the last two *orders* of the *class* 'universal diseases', 'dyspnoeas', includes all the breathing difficulties and is only indirectly associated with the nerves; the other, constituted by the 'mood disorders', occupies a rather peculiar place in MacBride's system. He accepted that there was an intimate association between mind and body but called into question the usefulness of carrying out physiopathological or anatomopathological studies: 'Albeit pathologists may be able to comment upon the disordered movements affecting those parts of the nervous system which are individually relevant to the internal senses, they cannot say much on the nature of their association...alterations found in the brain of dements constitute no more than objects of curiosity for they suggest little in the way of therapeutic implications...'[70] MacBride proposed however no alternative view and after dividing the mood disorders into two *genera*: 'mania' and 'melancholy' concluded that their analysis would be 'very complex'.

Under 'local diseases' he included conditions which could otherwise be classified as mood or nervous disorders such as morbid states affecting the external senses[71] and the appetites.[72] Particularly interesting is the *order* that includes the local alterations of the internal senses into which, together with amnesia and amentia, MacBride classified hypochondria which he considered as a 'disease of the imagination'. MacBride also commented upon the nosological distinctness of hysteria: 'Some feel that hysteria in women corresponds to hypochondria in men; this is not altogether correct for the hysterical temperament consists in hyperaesthesia with weakness of the solid parts and this gives rise to its variety of symptoms and forms'.[73]

One of the last attempts to utilize *more botanico* taxonomy in the English-speaking countries was made by John Mason Good in his *A Physiological System of Nosology*, published in London in 1817.[74] Basing his system on physiological principles, Good included six *orders* in his classification, each corresponding to alterations in one of the bodily functions: digestion, respiration, circulation and nervous, sexual and secretory. The resulting classification comprised the *orders*:

> 'I Coeliaca
> II Pneumatica
> III Haematica
> IV Neurotica
> V Genetica
> IV Eccritica'

'Neurotica' is defined as grouping 'diseases resulting from alteration of nervous function'. Good's effort was didactic but modest; in fact a number of his definitions are tautological.

Some British authors could be mentioned who included neither the term nor the concept 'Neurosis' in their work; this was the case of systems developed on speculative foundations.

Erasmus Darwin's *Zoonomia* (1796) and the surgical nosography (1825) by W. W. Sleigh[75] constitute good examples of this group. Brownism[76] however could be said to be the best historical illustration of a speculative pathology where the term neurosis is conspicuous by its absence. John Brown (1735–1788) was the creator of this system; a disciple of Cullen, he translated the work of his teacher into Latin and tutored his children; their relationship during later years however was soured by Brown's ungratefulness and his vehement attacks on the Scottish Professor. Brownism can be described as both a re-elaboration and a critique of Cullen's views. It is based on the premise that life is not an immanent property of the body but a 'forced state', that is, activity which results from and is driven by external stimuli. Brown grouped diseases in terms of two pathogenic principles: 'esthenia' or 'excessive excitement' and 'asthenia' or 'defective excitement' which may result either from absence of stimuli (direct asthenia) or from organismic fatigue consequential upon excessive stimuli (indirect asthenia). All clinical differentiations disappear into the simple dichotomic division of 'esthenic' and 'asthenic' diseases; and the Brownian clinician is only interested in measuring the level of 'excitement'. Brown therefore gave up diagnosis:

> Diagnosis is a relevant doctrine if it is assumed that there are many diseases as different amongst themselves as the names used for them...this work shows that this assumption is mistaken and that the infinite variety of diseases can be reduced to two forms, esthenic and asthenic, that differ only in level of excitement. The grand diagnostic textbooks have therefore become useless...and the work demanded from the physician superfluous...[77]

Neuroses therefore can hardly find a place in this system. Brown included mild hysteria, hypochondria, paralysis and tetanus in the group of severe asthenic diseases; mania and insomnia he considered as 'esthenic' diseases.

Brown's work highlights an important feature of the concept of neurosis, to wit, its dependence on clinical observation and inductive nosology. Perhaps because of its simplicity Brownism reached great popularity in Europe; for example it was considered as the medical doctrine of the future by the French Convention at the same level as Newton's ideas. With the exception of Great Britain, where it never caught on, all European countries developed Brownian groups. Heterodox Brownianism became one of the main sources of speculative medicine during the German Romanticism (so-called 'Naturphilosophie'). Likewise Brownian elements can be found in the view developed by the French physician Broussais, who was to exercise considerable influence on the development of the concept of neurosis.

The term and concept of neurosis were carried to the German-speaking countries[78] by the work of Cullen. The translation of his *First Lines of the Practice of Physick* went through three reprints,

Synopsis nosologiae through five, and the lectures on Neurosis through at least two. The word neurosis was translated as *Nervenkrankheit* ('nervous disease') and the literal rendition of this term was used in other languages.[79] Neurosis and nervous disease, therefore, should be considered as equivalent words until the early nineteenth century.[80]

The University of Göttingen was the German school more associated with British medicine and Cullen's work;[81] hence it is not surprising that it played an important role in the diffusion of the concept and term neurosis in Central Europe. Ernst Gottfried Baldinger, one of its main representatives, wrote a eulogy of Cullen's work, particularly of his nosological classification and Johann Heinrich Fischer published a scholarly account, his *Genera Morborum Cullenii* (1786).[82] Other works by the Göttingen school however did not include the concept of neurosis; instead they placed the various members of the group into different *classes* in the same way that they had been treated by pre-Cullean nosologies, such as that by R. A. Vogel, published in 1764. An example of this fragmentary view is constituted by Arnemann's book (1793) that keeps 'morbi spastici', the 'morbi a sensibilitate ac irritabilitate imminuta' and the 'Vesaniae'[83] as separate classes.

Christian Gottlieb Selle, another associate of the Göttingen school, also dealt with the concept of 'Nervous disease' in his *Rudimenta Pyretologiae* (1777) and *Medicina Clinica* (1781), both widely read in Europe.[84] Selle cultivated *more botanico* taxonomy which he based on what he called the analysis of the 'Nature of the disease'. He distinguished the 'causa materialis', that is, the ongoing pathological process affecting the 'solids or fluids' in the body from the 'causa formalis', that is, the particular disposition of the individual; the latter would explain why a 'causa materialis' may give rise to different symptomatology[85] in different individuals.

Selle did not consider pathological anatomy to be relevant to the description or identification of the 'causa materialis' (i.e. the 'nature of the disease') because he believed that, at its best, it would only uncover the superficial changes caused by the morbid process. He also regarded most symptoms as subjective and equivocal expressions of disease; more important were the 'indicantia', that is the symptoms that suggested treatment; a positive therapeutic response could, in turn, be used to clarify the 'nature of the disease'.[86]

When dealing with the concept of 'nervous disease' Selle stated in his *Medicina clinica*: 'Authors call "nervous diseases" or "of the nerves" those resulting from a direct affection of the nervous system leading to changes in sensitive and locomotor faculties';[87] he went on: 'Nervous diseases can be divided into two groups. One, of nervous diseases proper, results from marked weakness of the nervous system, in which case minor causes, insufficient to alter a normal constitution, may create havoc... the other comprises nerve disorders resulting from injury by major causes, which are able to hurt any constitution...'.[88]

Selle named the former 'morbi nervosi' and the latter 'morbi nervorum'. In his *Pyretologia* he defined 'morbi nervosi' aphoristically: 'symptoms (in this group) lack correspondence with one another and with their causes; there is a heightened sensitivity of mood and body'.[89] Two conclusions can be drawn from this definition: one that these conditions exhibit protean symptomatology; Selle put it this way: 'diseases in this class are characterized by irregular presentation of phenomena and causes';[90] the other, that the 'nature' of the neurosis (in Selle's terms the 'causa materialis') relates to the heightened sensitivity of the nervous system that renders it vulnerable to noxae. The conditions included by Selle amongst the 'morbi nervosi' vary from book to book. In *Pyretologia* three *genera* are included: '1. Morbi ex idiosyncrasia; 2. Morbi morales; and, 3. Malum hypochondriacum et hystericum'. His definition of the third genus tallies well with his general view of the 'morbi nervosi': 'The material cause resides in a nervous system that is weak and irritable';[91] but in his *Medicina clinica* Selle did not define 'nervous diseases' and only mentioned 'malum hypochondriacum et hystericum'.[92] Selle's work influenced the so-called 'First Berlin Medical School', an eclectic movement developed during the early nineteenth century of which Hufeland was the main exponent.

The Vienna School also came under the influence of Cullen during the last quarter of the eighteenth century which also corresponds to the second period of the *Alte Wiener Schule*. The views on nervous disease entertained in Vienna and in Göttingen during these years were similar in that some authors sponsored a fragmented, and others a unified, view of the nervous diseases. Johann Baptist Sagar amongst the former included the conditions usually grouped as neuroses into different classes; in his nosological system (1771) he considered 'dolores', 'anhelationes', 'spasmi', 'debilitates' and 'vesaniae' as independent classes.[93]

Johann Peter Frank amongst the latter made use of terms equivalent to 'nervous disease'. He was one of the initiators of public hygiene and made important contributions some of which will be mentioned later.[94] He wrote *De Curandis hominum morbis epitome* (1792–1821) whose innumerable editions and translations served as textbook to many European physicians; this book contains an excellent résumé of the view of neurosis held during the period prior to the development of the anatomoclinical method.[95] Frank disliked theoretical specula- tion and put emphasis on observation; he sponsored *more botanico* taxonomy but considered it to have only didactic value: 'Classifications add nothing to science but make it easier'.[96] This attitude also coloured his view on the 'neurosis', the seventh *class* of his system: 'So far we have not dealt with the various bodily systems in a separate fashion for this method is unhelpful; in the particular case of the nervous diseases, however because of their relevance and complexities...we shall do 'differently'.[97] The view contained in this quotation that the neuroses are an odd class has characterized these conditions since their inception and led many to believe that they may deserve a special place. But in Frank there is also present a complementary and rather novel view, namely that the neuroses are a provisional concept whose fate rests upon scientific progress: '...until such a time when we acquire a better knowledge of the human body, we are forced to accept the "nervous diseases".'[98]

The diffusion of the concept of neurosis in central-European medicine during this period was due not only to Göttingen and Vienna. Works published in other centres, representing varied theor- etical orientations, also contributed to this process. In this regard two books which include the term 'neurosis' will be mentioned: *Systema aegritudinum* (1781–1782) by Christian Friedrich Daniel, a physician from Halle and *Praxis medica* (1789) by Fredik Ludwig Bang, a Professor at Copenhagen; this latter work became well known through its German version (1791).

Daniel's book adopted the classical notions of 'nosos' and 'pathos' and distinguished three factors in the disease process: 'Morbi', 'passiones' and 'symptomata'. Guided by the 'symptomata' Daniel believed he could identify the basic 'passiones' that caused the 'morbi' or diseases. Neurosis he considered as one of the basic 'passiones' together with 'sepsis, saburra, plethora, pyogenia, catarrheuma, cachexia, conjunctio, dystrophia, ectopia' and an anonymous 'passio' reserved for unknown diseases.[99] The doctrine of humours also plays an important role in Daniel's work. It is of some interest therefore to notice that the concept of neurosis, whose links with modern views and traditional solidistic theory have already been commented upon, is reintroduced by Daniel but against the background of what can only be described as a speculative restatement of ancient medicine.

Bang's work, on the other hand, has only didactic pretensions. The Danish Professor adopted Cullen's classification as a theoretical framework within which to incorporate his rich clinical experience. He included five classes of disease: 'I – Pyrexiae; II – Dolores non febriles; III – Neuroses; IV – Morbi excretionum; and V – Cachexia'.

'Neuroses' or 'Nervenkrankheiten' mean in this classification basically the same as in Cullen's but are less dependent upon 'neuralpathology'. Three *genera* are included: 'adinamia or debility', 'spasmi' and 'madness'.[100]

The concept of neurosis gradually lost its 'neuralpathological' interpretation as it became assimilated into German medicine. To neuralpathology, writers like Frank, referred in unflattering terms 'to those who want to consider all diseases as nervous we leave the task of demonstrating the practical usefulness of so doing'.[101] And in cases when the 'Neuralpathological method' was partially adopted a rather peculiar view of the neuroses seemed to develop such as the one found in Gottfried Ploucquet, Professor at Tübingen; his conception of neurosis is worthy of attention as it contains the seeds of the various views which were to reign during the nineteenth century.

Ploucquet is well known for his bibliographical work on the medical literature of about the turn of the eighteenth century and also for the creation of a complex medical nomenclature which makes the reading of his work very laborious and which deprived him of any followers. A supporter of *more botanico* taxonomy he published *Delineatio systematis nosologica* (1791–1793) in an effort to develop a precise classificatory method.[102]

The two principles that inspired Ploucquet's nosology are 'the site or locus of the disorder' and the 'potential for injury'.[103] Precise knowledge on the two can be obtained in each clinical case from five sources: 'morbid praeternatural sensations', 'functional alterations', 'changes in sensible qualities', 'post-mortem data' and 'individual and occasional circumstances'.[104] Post-mortem studies are considered as particularly important in order to 'anchor abstract ideas on objective foundation' thereby 'doing away with subjectivity'.[105]

Ploucquet outlines *seven* classes:

      I Nevronusi (nervous diseases)
      II Peritropenusi (circulatory diseases)
      III Anapnoenusi (respiratory diseases)
      IV Trophonusi (nutritional diseases)
      V Ecrisionusi (excretion diseases)
      VI Genonusi (generative diseases)
      VII Alloeoses (mutation of sensible qualities)[106]

The term 'Nevronusi', derived from the Greek according to Ploucquet's personal rules, means 'nervous diseases'; but the author defined it no further. The *class* Nevronusi comprises six *orders*:

I Nevrastheniae (nervous weakness)
II Erethismi (irritations)
III Cinonusi (diseases of movement)
IV Aestheneatonusi (diseases of the senses and of sensory organs)
V Noonusi (mental diseases)
VI Mynopathi (sleep disorders)[107]

Ploucquet included 'fevers' and 'inflammations', whether acute or chronic, under 'Erethismi' and considered them to result from 'irritation'[108] of the nervous system (following the 'neuralpathology' of Cullen and Thaer). Ploucquet was also the first to utilize the term 'neurasthenia'. It will later be shown that the influence of 'neuralpathology' can also be detected in the work of Johann Christian Reil and that the concept of 'irritation' (as applied to neurosis) played a role in the development of Broussais's doctrine and in the creation of the concept of 'spinal irritation'.

The concept of neurosis fared differently in France than it did in Great Britain and central Europe. This may be explained by the fact that Pinel's *Nosographie philosophique* (1789) popularized the anatomoclinical view earlier in France than anywhere else. Pinel was also the first French translator of the work of Cullen (1785),[109] although Bosquillon's later version became better known.[110]

2: *The concept of neurosis in German romantic medicine*

Germany's odd position in European medicine during the early part of the nineteenth century stems partially from her support of romantic speculative medicine, or so-called *Naturphilosophie*, in a period during which other countries (e.g. Austria and Britain) had already adopted the anatomoclinical view initiated by the Paris school.

Therefore, before exploring the impact of the anatomoclinical view, an account will be given of the way in which the concept of neurosis was influenced by speculative pathology and by its rival doctrines. One of these was eclecticism and the other a collection of views that, after 1830, marked the transition from *Naturphilosophie* to the anatomopathological view.

Absence of the concept of neurosis in the work of the followers of 'Naturphilosophie'

Naturphilosophie refers to a complex speculative movement that developed in Germany during the romantic period out of the idealist philosophy of Schelling;[111] associated mainly with the southern German Universities, its sponsors produced numerous publications during the first three decades of the nineteenth century.

How important is *Naturphilosophie* to the historical study of the concept of neurosis? It could be speculated that the tendency amongst the romantics to 'personalize' nature – that led writers such as Ringseis to postulate a link between disease and sin – might also have affected the evolution of the neurosis, for example by suggesting a *sui generis* and personalized formulation of the concept. The search for historical precedence however is always a bad historiographic technique. In fact *Naturphilosophie* writers never 'anticipated' any of those current models that consider the neuroses as individualized disturbances. This lack of 'anticipation' can be

25

explained by the fact that the *Naturphilosophen* even more so than
the Brownians were remote from the clinical realities of inductivist
nosography. Thus it can be said that their highly speculative
methodology was blind to a concept that depends so much on clinical
observation: *Naturphilosophie* did not even oppose the concept; it
simply passed it by. Johann Nepomuk Ringseis' *System der Medizin*
(1841) illustrates this well[112] as it is one of the few books written by
Naturphilosophen to mention the term 'neurosis'. Ringseis listed the
concept *in passim* when criticizing various nosological systems based
on *more botanico* taxonomy; but while concepts such as *Morphen* or
Hämatosen deserved his critical attention, *Neurosen* did not in spite of
the fact that the term is present in at least eleven of the systems he
included (Cullen, Frank, Bang, Pinel, Daniel, Hufeland, Hildebrand,
Raimann, Ploucquet, Start and Schönlein).[113] Similar Olympian
disregard is shown by other *Naturphilosophen* and their classifications,
based on *a priori* speculative principles, could hardly entertain the
clinical concept of 'nervous disease'.

This uneasy interaction between the concept of neurosis and
Naturphilosophie continued even in the work of authors who were not
declaredly *Naturphilosophen* but who had some interest in speculative
philosophy. Amongst these the name of the vitalist physician Johann
Christian Reil, who ended up associating himself with *Naturphilosophie*,
should be mentioned; the so-called eclectics who criticized speculative
medicine from both traditional and modern vantage points, also dealt
with the concept of neurosis; and so did the generation led by Johann
Lucas Schönlein who served in Germany as a bridge between
romantic pathology and the anatomoclinical method. The evolution
of the concept of neurosis from Reil to Virchow cannot be traced
without taking into consideration these idealist efforts to understand
the nature of man and his diseases.

The concept of 'nervous disease' in Reil
The views of Johann Christian Reil (1759–1813), who shares with
Pinel the title of founder of Psychiatry, are important to the analysis
of German medicine during this period;[114] a comparison of the two
should illustrate major differences between German and French
medicine. Pinel represents a transitional stage between the Enlightenment and the new medicine and the view of neurosis he created lived

through the anatomoclinical period. Reil presided over the culmination of eighteenth century German medical vitalism and over its gradual transition to *Naturphilosophie* and eclecticism. Before undertaking the analysis of the concept of neurosis developed by Reil in *Ueber Erkenntnis und Kur der Fieber* (1800–15)[115] a brief account will be given of other relevant aspects of his thought.

A strong Kantian influence allowed Reil to assimilate the medical views sponsored during this period by the medical schools of Göttingen and Halle; he also applied Kant's theory of knowledge to the study of disease and to the basic principles of his vitalist doctrine.[116]

Reil rejected the theoretical 'panneurogenism' of 'neuralpathology' although he was prepared to entertain the view that the nervous system may exert some influence on the rest of the organs:

> There is no reason to consider all disorders of the body as
> nervous diseases for they may be only secondarily causing a
> nervous ailment; it is true, of course, that on occasions
> changes in the nervous system may cause alterations
> elsewhere; but in neither case should what obtains be called
> nervous disease for the location of the phenomena in
> question is not in the nerves themselves but in other parts of
> the body...[117]

This quotation indicates that Reil (like other writers) believed that the neuroses held a simple relationship to the nervous system and disregarded any 'special relationship' of a conceptual kind such as the one postulated by 'neuralpathology'. The same cannot be said of his view on other morbid conditions however as his concept of 'fever' for example contained remnants of 'neuralpathology'.

Reil was a supporter of *more botanico* taxonomy. In *Ueber Erkenntnis und Kur der Fieber*, he stated the wish to 'outline a natural system for the theory of fevers'; enterprise which he compared with the work of a botanist.[118] His taxonomic ontologism led him to consider *genera* and *species* as ontologically real but '*classes* and *orders* as man made and not necessarily based on reality'.[119] He dismissed symptoms, aetiologies and even Selle's 'indicantia' as of little classificatory value. Instead he based his classification, rather imprecisely, on disease locus and patient's biotype: 'Is there an identifiable organic alteration? of what organ? how is the resulting morbid state modified by the patient's constitution? The answers to these questions should provide us with full knowledge of the disease. They may be abstract questions but provide the key for a (nosological) system'.[120]

The five volumes of *Ueber Erkenntnis und Kur der Fieber* took a number of years to be published and the last volume, edited by Christian Friedrich Nasse, appeared posthumously. This fifth volume includes much information on the pathological knowledge of the period and is dedicated to Reil's view on 'fever'. Under this category an unusual number of morbid states are included such as fevers proper, inflammation and congestion, haemorrhages, exanthematas, glandular disorders and the 'nervous diseases'. On the origin of this over-encompassing view Neuburger has written thus:

> The peculiar Reilian theory of fever is already contained in
> his *Memorabilia clinica*. It originates from the observation
> that fever is usually accompanied by disordered (increased)
> activity in many organs; Reil believed that this augmented
> activity did not only stem from the excitement generated by
> the fever but from alterations in vitality which, in the last
> analysis, had to be explained as resulting from abnormal
> composition of the organs. By focusing his attention on
> 'local' fever, ondulant fever affecting isolated parts of the
> body, inflammation etc. Reil concluded that heightened
> organic activity and irritability were the essence of fever.
> And by considering 'functional capacity' as the second
> defining factor he identified two species of fever: 'Synocha'
> and 'Typhus'. The inclusion of two other clinical
> observations, namely, weakness and paralysis (often present
> in malignant fever) led him to describe a third species
> 'Paralysis' (Lähmung)....[121]

According to Reil all 'fevers' are *dynamic* in nature: 'A fever consists in a praeternatural alteration of the animal forces and a heightened irritability leading to reduced functional capacity without appreciable structural change and to increased irritability in the vessels and nerves associated with the affected organ'.[122] But not all 'fevers' are *general*: 'fever is not necessarily general nor is it specifically associated with a given organ; indeed it may affect any of them'.[123]

Reil's inclusion of the neuroses under the category 'fever' and also his classification of the fevers must be understood against the context of Cullen's influence and in relation to his partial acceptance of 'neuralpathology'; this theoretical position was similar to that taken by other authors such as Ploucquet during this period.

'A disease of the nerves' Reil defined as: 'an abnormal vital process leading to an alteration in the known properties and functions of the nerves'.[124] This tautological definition reflects the fundamental difficulty bedevilling the notion of nervous disease, namely that the only available background against which to define these conditions is the nervous system. Pinel, in an attempt to break the circle added a second criterion: absence of anatomopathological lesion.[125] For Reil, however, the anatomoclinical view was no more than a quest for anatomical localization and never possessed the conceptual importance it had for the French author. Hence Reil's formulations and classification remained at the localizationistic level.

Reil's view of the neuroses is in keeping with these principles. On proximal causes he wrote:

> What is usually considered as a proximal cause of nervous disease is either a groundless hypothesis or a remote cause. Some authors seem to believe that alterations of the nervous humour amount to a proximal cause, however the very existence of this humour and of its secretion by the brain can be called into question... other authors refer instead to relaxation, loss of tone or rigidity or dryness of the nerves or occlusion of its covering... (however) the proximal cause of nervous disease (or what is the same, the nervous disease itself) should be sought in the disorders affecting the dynamics and the constituent matter of the nervous system, in which I include not only the nerves but also their vascular membranes.[126]

Reil defined the neuroses in terms of his dynamic view of 'fever' but also considered them as localized alterations of the nervous system; for him the neuroses are *dynamic* disorders but no longer *general*; he therefore can be said to do away with all vitalistic explanations. This would seem to justify the view that Reil was a transitional author. His transitional character is also reflected in his classification of the neuroses or 'Nervenkrankheiten'. Although basing it on observed symptoms he sought a degree of anatomical localization: '1. Diseases of the coenesthesia; 2. Diseases of the organs of external senses; 3. Diseases of the internal senses; 4. Diseases characterized by abnormal sympathy; 5. Diseases of the nerves associated with vegetative life'.[127]

The concept of neurosis in the work of Christoph Wilhelm Hufeland and of other eclectic authors

Christoph Wilhelm Hufeland (1762–1836) is the most important representative of the group of German physicians that defended an eclectic viewpoint and opposed *Naturphilosophie* during the first half of the nineteenth century. His work served as a link between the school of Göttingen, heir to the Hallerian tradition, and the new school of Berlin, that was to be so important in the future.[128]

Hufeland never studied in Paris and had only a limited and indirect knowledge of the new anatomoclinical method. Nonetheless he supported clinical observation and common sense against the speculative excesses of *Naturphilosophie*, Brownism, homeopathy, mesmerism etc. His heterogeneous doctrine was predominantly vitalistic but with a sprinkling of the anatomoclinical method and even with the occasional reference to the speculative doctrines he antagonized. His clinical orientation is reflected in the way he formulated a diagnosis:

> The first condition for treatment is knowledge of the disease.
> But, what does this knowledge consist of? It cannot be
> limited to the name of the disease or to its external
> manifestations (i.e. to achieving nominal, historicocultural or
> nosological diagnosis) for this information can only lead to
> external, superficial and symptomatic treatment; the
> knowledge of the disease must include the causative morbid
> state. Only knowledge of this kind can lead to real
> treatment...we call it practical diagnosis...i.e. knowledge of
> the internal morbid state and its localization...but this must
> also include information on the person himself, on the
> suffering patient....[129]

This interest in the suffering patient led Hufeland to attach relevance to constitutional and hereditary factors and to consider systematic nosology as a mere framework within which clinical phenomena could be classified and interpreted from a vitalist perspective.

In his *Enchiridion medicum* (1836) Hufeland developed a classification that included thirteen classes and two special categories
dedicated to diseases of women and children. One of the *classes*,
'neurosis', he defined as 'disordered activity (disease) of sensibility,
movement or mind which must be idiopathic or primary to the
nervous system and not a mere symptom of other disease or if
secondary to other disease must appear as a pure disease of the
nervous system'.[130] This definition, reminiscent of Cullen's, introduces
an interesting distinction between idiopathic and symptomatic
neuroses. In general Hufeland's definition is clinically more precise
than the schematic notion of the Scottish physician. This allows him
to identify a number of clinical aspects such as the unpredictable
evolution and uncertain outcome; the protean quality of the symptoms
and the facility with which they may change into one another.[131]
Together with Hufeland's 'practical' vein other conceptual influences
also shaped his work on the neuroses. For example vitalism influenced
his pathogenic view: 'the proximal cause refers to an abnormal state
of internal nervous life manifesting itself in unusual behaviour and
in morbid changes in organic life...'[132]

In general eclectic writers suffered from a lack of conceptual
solidity which on occasions led them to accept viewpoints taken from
speculative medicine; this might explain why Hufeland made use of
Brown's notion of 'asthenia'. Writing on the origin of nervous
'weakness' he concluded: 'It may result from lack of stimuli and of
vital substances, deficiency or bad quality of nutrition, pernicious or
"animalized" air, lack of heat..., menstrual loss, excessive seminal
loss, chronic loss of serum or mucus, diarrhoea, *fluor albus*..., or
from overstimulation and exhaustion, psychical or muscular fatigue
and febrile and chronic diseases...'[133]

The response of Hufeland to the influence of the anatomoclinical
method is partial and hesitating, but more decisive than the imprecise
localizationism of Reil's. The anatomical lesion criterion allowed
Hufeland to write: 'when dealing with a nervous disease the first
question must be: is it a disease with material basis, in other words
is it a nervous disease or does it result from a lesion elsewhere in the
body?'[134] The former, which, according to Hufeland, were caused by
a dynamic alteration of the 'nervous life', he called idiopathic
neurosis; the latter he referred to as symptomatic neuroses and

related to *materielle Fehler*. This distinction is based, albeit incompletely, on anatomoclinical assumptions.

Hufeland also considered – as Selle had done before him – *Nervöse Constitution* to be a predisposing factor in the development of the neuroses. Temporarily lost during the anatomoclinical period, this view re-emerged during the latter part of the nineteenth century.

Ludwig Wilhelm Sachs, Professor of Medicine at Koenigsberg, was a disciple of Hufeland's.[135] In his *Handbuch des natürlichen Systems der praktischen Medizin* (1828) Sachs supported the eclectic view of his teacher, opposing the speculative medicine of *Naturphilosophie* and emphasizing the need to free the experimental sciences from metaphysics.[136] His ideas, based on clinical observation, he sought to complement by anatomical and physiological research and post-mortem data. In spite of its empirical foundations Sachs's work shows speculative features which may find at least partial origin in the vitalism of the Enlightenment; another speculative influence on Sachs was the system developed by Karst, following Fichte's idealist philosophy.

Karst's notion of disease was based on the idealist opposition between man as an 'individual' and nature as a 'totality'. Disease resulted from the struggle between two antagonistic forces, 'Autokratie' and 'Physiokratie'; the former maintaining individuality, the latter the unity of nature. The struggle is enacted in all three organic systems: nervous or sensitive, irritable and vegetative or reproductive.[137]

Sachs's systematic nosology is based upon the resulting dynamic interactions in the three organic systems. He identified three 'Haupklassen': inflammation ('Entzündung'), fever ('Fieber') and neurosis ('Nervenkrankheiten').

Inflammation results from attempts by the organism to protect its integrity in all three organic systems.[138] Fever, on the other hand is defined as a response to external stimuli that manifests itself only in the irritable system.[139]

The third *class*, the neuroses, is characterized by organismic changes which depend upon the quality and not the intensity of the stimulus. The *class* neuroses is subdivided into *orders* corresponding to diseases of 'organic excitation' and of the 'spirit and mood'.[140] In spite of his efforts to move away from *Naturphilosophie*, Sachs's view of the neurosis remained aprioristic and little connected with clinical observation.

Eclectic writers without the personality of Hufeland and with less desire to speculate than Sachs, limited themselves to repeating doctrines from the latter part of the eighteenth century; amongst these Johann Valentin von Hildenbrand and Johann Nopomuk von Raimann could be mentioned; their work can be regarded as transitional between the 'alte' and the 'neue Wiener Schule'.

Hildenbrand attempted, in his *Institutiones medico-practicae* (1816–1825), to develop a 'system free from speculation'; in the end he just managed to repeat, although without its terminological complexity, the classification proposed by Franz X. Schwediaur or Swediauer, a Viennese physician trained in Edinburgh. Hildenbrand considered five *classes*:

1. Fevers
2. Caquexias
3. Neuroses
4. Secretions
5. Local diseases[141]

The *class* Neuroses 'included diseases resulting from alterations in the function, forces and faculties of the nervous system (apart from fevers) such as pain-producing disorders, diseases of the mind and movement, hyperaesthesias, spasms, respiratory difficulties, weakness and vesanias'.[142] The strong Cullean influence showed by this definition was transmitted to Hildenbrand by Swediauer and Frank.

A similar comment can be made on the view of neurosis expressed in Raimann's *Handbuch der speziellen medizinischen Pathologie und Therapie* (1815–1817): 'Neuroses or nervous diseases, sensu stricto, are disorders of isolated nerves or of the nervous system as a whole, which manifest themselves primarily and mainly as alterations of external or internal senses, disorders of muscular movement or both.'[143]

Ernst von Grossi trained in Vienna but spent his professional life in Bavaria, one of the centres of *Naturphilosophie*. Like Hildenbrand and Raimann, he adopted Enlightenment ideas to oppose speculative medicine; his *Opera medica posthuma* (1831) contains one of the most complicated classifications ever published. Neuroses are included in eight different *classes*:

XXX Cineses
XXXI Discineses
XXXII Aesthesiae
XXXIII Dysaestesiae
XXIV Epithymiae
XXXV Aversationes
XXXVI Hyperaesthematospasmi
XXXVII Narco-Anaestheseospasmi[144]

This baroque terminology tells little more than the author's view that the neuroses are alterations of motility, sensibility and mind.

Baldinger's views (mentioned above) were continued in Göttingen up to the middle of the nineteenth century by Johann Wilhelm Heinrich Conradi. From an eclectic viewpoint this writer opposed both speculative medicine and the transitional views of Schoenlein and Broussais. His *Specielle Pathologie* (1811) allocates neuroses to five different *classes*:

VII Pain
VIII Aberrant and exaggerated sensations
IX Adynamiae
X Spasmi
XI Mental Diseases[145]

A last illustration of the views on neurosis entertained by the German eclectic school is Johann Ludwig Choulant's *Lehrbuch der speciellen Pathologie und Therapie des Menschen* (1831). Although mainly remembered for his historical work Choulant was a remarkable clinician of vitalist persuasion. His classification is based on the traditional distinction between vital, natural and animal functions:

I Diseases of the vital functions:	fevers, inflammations and congestions
II Diseases of the reproductive functions:	disorders of excretion, secretion, neoformations and consumption
III Diseases of the animal functions:	nervous and mental diseases, ecliptic states[146]

Choulant managed to reduce the number of diseases considered as neuroses or 'Nervenkrankheiten' but not to the extent achieved by the French anatomoclinicians. Choulant included twelve morbid species in his group:

1 Thoracic spasm in the adult
2 Thoracic spasm in children
3 Nightmares
4 Formication
5 *Delirium Tremens*
6 Paralysis
7 Apoplexy
8 Tonic convulsions
9 Epilepsy
10 St. Vito's dance
11 Hysteria
12 Hypochondria.[147]

The concept of neurosis during the transition between romantic and anatomoclinical medicine: Johann Lucas Schönlein and his school

The transition from romantic to scientifico–natural medicine took place in Germany after 1830 and was presided over by the physiologist Johannes Müller and the pathologist and internist Johann Lucas Schönlein (1793–1864). Brought up as a *Naturphilosoph*, Schönlein came to adopt the anatomoclinical principles[148] during his maturity; between these two end points, his work went through a number of transitional states. His disciples separate, according to the period they made contact with Schönlein, into an early 'parasitical' group, who still emphasized speculation; a 'historiconatural' group that continued cultivating *more botanico* taxonomy; and a 'scientifico-natural' group that assumed a clear anatomoclinical orientation. The way in which the concept of neurosis fared in relation to Schönlein's transitional views and to the various scientificonatural formulations of his school will now be explored.

Schönlein's publications on the neurosis are not numerous. Two of these, the lecture notes of Zürich (1839) and the *Klinische Vorträge*, given at the Charité in Berlin (1842)[149] are particularly illuminating. Schönlein's decision to disown the transitional view he expressed in the lecture notes was due less to any inexactitudes he might have detected in the transcription collated by his disciples than to the growth of his own thinking.

Schönlein's work contains at this stage three well-balanced components: *Naturphilosophie*, *more botanico* taxonomy and pathological anatomy. All three show well in his view on health and disease and in his classification:

> Healthy is the organism whose functions maintain a state of regularity both in the individual and in his species...Disease, as a negation of health, refers to a state of the organism in which dysfunction leads to loss of regularity in the individual and in his species. The concepts of health and disease are therefore opposite although...both constitute historiconatural phenomena that can only find expression in the course of organic life. From this it can be concluded that:
>
> 1. Being disease a characteristic of individuals and species, only organic systems can become diseased;
> 2. Being disease a manifestation of life, only living systems can become diseased; and,
> 3. Only organs and isolated systems can become diseased, never the totality of the organism. There can only be localized disease, for if all systems went wrong at the same time, the organism would change into something else and the individual and the species would disappear.[150]

This quotation shows Schönlein, at this stage of his development, combining pathological anatomy and speculative medicine. The speculative dimension is even more salient in the distinction he made between 'Morphonosen', 'Hämatonosen' and 'Neuronosen', adopting the vegetative, animal and sensitive principles of Schelling's philosophy.[151] But the most striking example of speculation is provided by his view on the ego-planet opposites:

> Medicine is about life in general and man in particular. Although part of the whole, man endeavours to achieve full independence; nature, however, has the tendency to engulf man. Whereupon an opposition develops between ego and the planetary force. For as long as the ego predominates, the planetary force is kept at bay and the being preserves its

independence (health)...but the predominance of the planetary force means death to the individual. Disease is the struggle between ego (independent life) and the planetary force (the noxious principle that threatens life).[152] Pathological anatomy was another foundation of Schönlein's nosology. During this early period he also adopted *more botanico* taxonomy; which was to be taken to extremes by the 'historiconatural' branch of his school. In his Zürich lectures Schönlein said: 'It is incumbent upon us to organize all known diseases into a system. Nosological, like botanical systems can be artificial or natural...'[153] Artificial systems are organized on the basis of 'a given feature of the array such as tooth or claws structure in certain animals...'[154]; artificial nosologies follow criteria such as: 'a capite ad calces', duration of the disease, chemical principles, and physiological principles which tend to 'neglect pathological anatomy'.[155] In opposition to artificial ones, 'natural systems are not based on a particular feature but on a set of fundamental manifestations. The first to attempt such a system was the Swiss physician F. Platter in 1677 (sic) (in original) and after him Sydenham, Linné and Cullen...'[156]

Schönlein dedicated a great deal of attention to Pinel's classification and to its anatomoclinical foundations[157] and confronted the negative criticisms levelled against systematic nosology: 'Of late some have considered all attempts to develop natural systems as useless. However, since this kind of work has been so successful in other natural sciences and since the current accumulation of facts demands it, it would not seem altogether pointless to try it again'.[158]

Schönlein suggested that previous classificatory efforts had failed through neglect of the anatomical lesion and an inadequate use of clinical symptomatology and attempted to put this right by assessing the nosological value of symptoms and seeking correlations with post-mortem data. The nosological method ('genetische Methode'), which in due course influenced so much the development of German medicine, was the outcome of this work.

The concept of neurosis developed by Schönlein in the Zürich lectures is based on a combination of romantic speculation, pathological anatomy and ontological nosology. He classified diseases according to the speculative distinction between vegetative, animal

and sensitive life and regarded the 'neuroses' or 'neuronosis' as
physiological alterations of sensitive life which are:

1. Localized in the nervous system. Hence, universal nervous
   diseases like general alterations of the blood are a contradiction
   in terms. Disorders of the nervous system are regional and affect
   separate systems such as the cerebral, spinal or ganglionar
   ones.
2. The functional alteration of the diseased part may be quan-
   titative, qualitative or both.
3. The resulting symptoms exhibit a degree of periodicity and
   symmetry.
4. Blood disorders are not qualitative but accidental and quan-
   titative in nature,...the same holds for secretions and
   excretions.
5. Temperature is reduced in most cases of neuroses; increased
   temperature is only accidental and temporary...[159]

These five points illustrate Schönlein's extremely localizationist
concept of the neuroses which he combined with views taken from
Naturphilosophie such as the 'symmetrical' character of the symptoms.
The neuroses he subdivided into:

1. Somatic neuroses, resulting from alterations of nervous activity
   inasmuch as this affects organic life.
2. Psychical neuroses – resulting from alterations of nervous
   activity inasmuch as this affects psychical life.[160]

Schönlein did not dedicate equal time to both. The 'psychical
neuroses' he dispatched quickly: 'Almost always the psychical
diseases, called by us psychical neuroses are based on some somatic
alteration; hence they can be explained away in terms of this material
basis'.[161]

'Somatic neuroses', on the other hand, are dealt with in extenso
and subdivided into three families:

(a) 'Intermittent neuroses' – which are differentiated from the
    'intermittent fevers' of old by the deletion of the word 'fever',
    thereby emphasizing their hypothetical nervous origin.[162]
(b) 'Neuralgias' – that include the 'spasmi' and 'pains' of old,
    which are rejected as subjective and lacking in definition.[163]
(c) 'Neuroses' proper, characterized by:

1. Peripheral localization of the morbid process. Centrally localized neuroses are not possible...
2. An episodic course, in which, however, the paroxysms are neither regular nor typical...
3. An excitation generated in the peripheral nervous system which, during the paroxysmal stage, reaches the central areas...
4. Isolated paroxysmal episodes which manifest themselves as spasmi and seizures...
5. Nervous activity, particularly perception, may be disordered or normal, heightened or damped down...[164]

The influence of ontological nosology and *more botanico* taxonomy is clear in the Lecture Notes. The old classificatory labyrinth is still present although modified by anatomopathological criteria which in the event led to the localizationist interpretation of the concept of neurosis. The 'general' character of the neuroses is thus lost in the work of Schönlein as it was amongst the French anatomoclinicians; Schönlein however was more radical than his teachers, as converts often are. The French anatomoclinicians' attempts to define the neuroses in terms of specific and constant anatomical lesions led to the paradoxical consequences that those morbid conditions in which a lesion was identified lost their character of neuroses. This negative consequence resulted from the fact that, since the times of Pinel, French anatomoclinicians had also defined the neuroses as conditions not accompanied by specific lesions. During his Zürich period, however, Schönlein accepted the view that the neuroses must be accompanied by anatomical lesions; after acknowledging that information was often scanty, Schönlein was still prepared to marshal opinion on the lesions that might be present in each 'neurosis'. Schönlein's transitional view therefore led him to sponsor a positive anatomopathological view of the neuroses. The scientificonatural branch of his school retained this view until it was superseded during the anatomoclinical period.

Of less historical interest is the group of Schönlein's disciples who supported the 'parasitical' view of disease. Karl Wilhelm Stark, under the influence of Dietrich Georg Kieser and borrowing speculative elements from Schönlein's earlier thinking, believed that diseases inhabited the affected organism and were endowed with independent existence. In his *Allgemeine Pathologie* (1838) he put forward a classification fashioned after the idea of a 'kingdom' of historico-natural species, one of which, 'neurosis', was the *class* associated with alterations of sensitive life.[165]

The 'historiconatural' branch of Schönlein's school adopted the formulation of the neurosis developed in the Zürich Lectures. Gottfried Eisenmann, one of its members, presented in his *Die vegetativen Krankheiten und die entgiftende Heilmethode* (1835) a nosological system including three *classes* resulting from alterations, respectively, in anatomical form ('Morphosen'), vegetative function ('Phytosen') and 'spiritual and sensitive life' ('Neurosen'). The speculative content of Eisenmann's views should not be allowed to conceal the fact that he expanded Schönlein's views on *more botanico* taxonomy. Attempting a 'natural classification' he subdivided the *class* 'neurosis' into:

Order 1: 'Vegetoneurosen'
Order 2: 'Neurosen' *sensu stricto*
    Family 1: 'Parapathien'
    Family 2: 'Parakinesen'
    Family 3: 'Parästhesien'
Order 3: 'Somatopsychrosen'
Order 4: 'Psychrosen'[166]

The term 'Psychrosen' included the mental diseases and replaced the old one of 'Geisteskrankheiten', which Eisenmann considered unacceptable on the argument that illness can only affect organic tissue but never the spirit (*Geist*) itself. He was critical of Ringseis and Heinroth, the main psychiatric writers of the *Naturphilosophie* movement.[167]

Joseph Friedrich Sobernheim, another of Schönlein's disciples, also followed the 'historiconatural' orientation; keener on pathological anatomy than Eisenmann, he defined the neuroses in his *Praktische Diagnostik der inneren Krankheiten* (1837) as 'pathological states sited in the nervous system where they primarily originate'.[168] After agreeing with Reil that knowledge on the nervous system was scanty he endeavoured to develop a classification of the neuroses based on anatomy and physiology:

1. Neurosis of the psychical activity and of the organs of the senses.
2. Neurosis of the sensitivity and of the organic movements.
3. Neurosis of the organs, that is, of the brain, spinal cord and ganglionar system.[169]

In spite of his efforts Sobernheim was unable to go beyond the eighteenth century nosologies:

> The symptoms of the nervous conditions manifest themselves from the phenomenological viewpoint as pathological sensations (algias), pathological movements (spasms) and perversions of behaviour (alienations, 'intemperantia nervorum'). Pathological sensations can be increased (hyperaesthesia) or decreased (anaesthesia), these two states corresponding to nervous inflammation (neuroflogosis) and nervous paralysis (neuroparalysis), respectively. Pathological movements find expression in muscle spasm characterized by contraction alone (tonic spasm) or by alternating contraction and relaxation (clonic spasm). Perversions of behaviour manifest themselves in pathological dysphoria (cravings, impulses, passions, abnormal sensations and behaviour) or in the development of morbid associations between secretory function and its pathological products, such as occurs in hypochondria, hysteria or diabetes...[170]

The 'scientificonatural' branch of Schönlein's school retained the positive lesion view of the neurosis until it was ready to accept the anatomoclinical view. The *Handbuch der medizinischen Klinik* (1843–1854) by Karl Canstatt, one of Schönlein's late disciples,[171] is a good example of this in that the anatomoclinical view inspires its attempts to explain nosological entities in terms of specific and localized anatomical lesions. However when dealing with the concept of neurosis the *Handbuch* shows the same level of uneasiness that was later to characterize the work of the French anatomoclinicians. Canstatt considered the neurosis as a woolly concept only retained by habit:

> to define neurosis or nervous disease is as difficult as defining vegetative disease..., the term neurosis is employed

when phenomena resulting from altered nervous life are met with. The neuroses constitute formal types or manifestations of diverse morbid processes. (Hence) the neuroses... may show similar manifestations even when the underlying primary states are different. Thus Epilepsy may be produced by a growth in a peripheral nerve or by the presence of worms; Tetanus may result from a peripheral nerve lesion, strychnine poisoning or an inflammation of the spinal cord. Albeit resulting from varied aetiology the neuroses can be said to have identical surface manifestations.[172]

Canstatt remained faithful to the view that the neuroses are accompanied by a specific lesion. As 'proximal causes' for these conditions he mentioned anatomical alterations such as hyperaemia, inflammation, scroffula and tumours.[173] By considering the neuroses as an ill-defined group of 'clinical manifestations' Canstatt avoided, as Schönlein had done before him, the problem of having to ascertain the presence of specific lesions in each case. His work, characterized by a timid application of pathological anatomy, should be considered as the final stage of the transitional period. In the complementary volume of Canstatt's *Handbuch* (1854), published posthumously, E. H. Henoch, its editor, abandoned Schönlein's ideas in favour of the French anatomoclinical view:

> What does the concept of neurosis refer to? The answer nowadays is even more difficult than it was in Canstatt's time... no other condition exemplifies better the usefulness of the pathological anatomy method, namely... that since no structural alteration can be detected by our senses in relation to the neuroses, a definition may not be possible. By 'nervous disease', therefore we mean states associated with functional alteration of the nervous system in relation to which no structural change has yet been described.[174]

The volume dedicated to the diseases of nervous system in the new *Handbuch* edited by Virchow appeared a year later. K. E. Hasse, its author,[175] declared: 'These diseases can be divided into two classes, one comprising the nervous diseases proper (neuroses) with no organic alteration; the other including cases of real alteration in the organs of the nervous activity'.[176]

The books by Henoch and Canstatt, by making a clear distinction between neurological disease and neurosis, acted as a bridge between the *Handbuch* of Canstatt, last representative of the old view, and the work of Virchow, first manifestation of the new period. They bring to a close an important era in the history of the concept of neurosis within German medicine.

3: *The concept of neurosis in anatomoclinical medicine before Charcot*

The anatomoclinical view provided the earliest conceptual foundation of scientificonatural medicine during the nineteenth century. This achievement of the anatomoclinicians Laín Entralgo has called the 'copernican revolution operated by the concept of anatomopathological lesion' for the anatomical lesion, until then less important than the symptom, became the very basis of medicine.[177]

A confrontation therefore was inevitable between the new view, based on *localization* and a *reduction to the anatomical level*, and the concept of neurosis, related since its inception to *general* diseases and interpreted *physiologically*. This confrontation will be explored first in the work of Pinel who presided over the transition between the Enlightenment and the new views; then in relation to the period during which efforts were made to jettison the concept of neurosis culminating with Georget's fundamental revision; finally its evolution will be traced during the zenith of the anatomoclinical view, between Georget and Charcot.

Pinel's work as the starting point of the anatomoclinical view of the neuroses

Paris was the indisputable capital of anatomoclinical medicine during the early nineteenth century. The French revolution and the ensuing sociopolitical climate had done away with all existing medical institutions and brought into being new ones free from the burden of tradition. For about twenty years Philippe Pinel (1745–1826), imbued by the ideal of a new medicine, presided over the transformation. Remembered as one of the founders of psychiatry, it is less known that he also forged the link between the Enlightenment and anatomoclinical pathology.[178]

Three themes from the Enlightenment are present in Pinel's work: *more botanico* taxonomy, vitalism, and the ideal of medicine as a

44

natural science. He did not limit himself, however, to the mechanical application of the botanical method as had been the case with Sauvages and followers. Pinel's ambition is well expressed in Bichat's view that medicine should be made into an 'exact science'; like Bichat and Laennec he resorted to pathological anatomy only when *more botanico* taxonomy required objective foundations but, in general, followed a 'via media' and did not subordinate clinical symptomatology to pathological anatomy. Pinel used Condillac's 'analytical method' less to explore morphology and semiology than to give an account of human disease as a 'vital response'. The transitional role played by Pinel's system is well illustrated in his choice of 'Primitive disease' as the notional counterpart for the 'simple idea' concept of Condillac's. This concept is neither Barthez's 'morbid element' nor Bichat's 'tissue' nor Laennec's 'auscultatory sound' but something in between, a sort of basic reality, stemming from both clinical and anatomopathological observation. As 'primitive diseases' he considered *fever, phlegmasia, haemorrhage, organic lesion* and *neurosis*. This is the starting point of his *Nosographie Philosophique*, published in 1798, soon abridged and translated into most European languages.[179] Pinel replaced the old classificatory principles of Sauvages's and Selle's by the 'happy idea of basing the classification of diseases on anatomical structure'.[180] The application of the principle, on occasions unproblematic, led to his analysis of the *phlegmasias* that was to serve as a model for Bichat's 'general anatomy'; in other cases however it was difficult or impossible: this forced Pinel to include a final class on *organic lesions* which he vaguely considered as 'associated with the preceding ones'. This hesitating and transitional classificatory view is also illustrated by his treatment of the neuroses.

Pinel did not provide a definition of these conditions. He simply described them as alterations of sensitivity and motility which are not accompanied by primitive fever, inflammation and structural lesion.[181] The superficial similarity of this definition to Cullen's, misled some of his followers into considering Cullen's 'morbi locales' as equivalent to Pinel's 'organic lesions'.

Pinel acknowledged that the 'Nervous diseases' had already been well studied by Whytt, Lorry, Pomme, etc. during the latter half of the eighteenth century and noticed that, according to their view, the main characteristic of these conditions was their protean clinical presentation. Pinel however did not resort to clinical presentation when outlining the *neuroses* as 'primitive diseases'; instead he defined them as alterations of 'sense' and 'movement': 'The difficulties posed by the description of the various nervous alterations of hearing, eyesight and other senses, of the various types of spasm, muscular convulsions, and of the Vesaniae and neuralgic pains, disappear when these conditions are considered as alterations of sense and movement'.[182] Pinel believed that the understanding of the neurosis should depend upon the obtention of scientific knowledge on these two vital phenomena: 'The description of the nervous diseases, that is of the pathological conditions of the nervous function which are not accompanied by fever or phlegmasia, must be based upon the information that physiological research is offering us on sense and movement...'[183] Pinel's realization that the anatomoclinical view was not sufficient did not lead however to a fuller development of the physiopathological view. Gaps in physiological knowledge were still too wide and in the end Pinel limited himself to a pure description of the phenomena.[184] In fact, a considerable time had to elapse before medical thinking came to regard physiopathology as a possible solution to the conundrum of the neurosis. All Pinel could do was to resort to the stock reference to the nervous system which he conceals under the new terminology:

> The many functional alterations found in the neuroses constitute in spite of their variety, a class of disorders which is closely associated with the nervous system. This system commences in the encephalus, spreads out to all parts of the body, and transmits sense and movement to activate the organic functions.[185]

The novel feature in Pinel's view is his exclusion of the 'structural lesion' principle. However, the general drift of his argument is contradicted by his claim that anatomical lesions can cause certain neuroses. This contradiction he tried to resolve by considering these neuroses as 'symptomatic' and not as neuroses proper.[186] Along the same lines he wrote on the 'organic lesions', the last *class* of his system: 'For as long as the neuroses remain unchanged and are not accompanied by degeneration of the tissues involved, it can be said that they constitute that class of diseases whose characteristics have already been mentioned'.[187] Pinel's vacillations should not obscure the fact that it is in his work that the 'principle of negative lesion', basic feature of the anatomoclinical period, is for the first time clearly linked to the concept of neuroses.

A consequence of this new view was a progressive reduction in the number of neuroses which resulted from the elimination of those conditions in which a specific lesion was found. In spite of this, Pinel collected in his *class* 'neurosis' a number as high as Cullen's. His classification in the *Nosographie Philosophique* is as follows:

Order I Neuroses of the senses
    of hearing: deafness; paracusia; tinnitus etc.
    of vision: diplopia; hemeralopia; amaurosis etc.
Order II Neuroses of cerebral function
    comas: apoplexy; catalepsy; epilepsy
    Vesaniae: hypochondria; melancholia; mania; amentia;
      idiocy; hydrophobia etc.
Order III Neuroses of the organs of locomotion and of the voice
    of locomotion: neuralgia; tetanus; convulsions; chorea;
      palsy
    of voice: convulsive voice; aphonia
Order IV Neuroses of nutrition
    of digestion: dysphagia; cardialgia; pyrosis; spasmodic
      vomiting; bulymia; pica; dyspepsia; anorexia; nervous
      colic etc.
    of breathing: asthma; asphyxia; whooping cough
    of circulation: nervous palpitations; sincope
Order V Neuroses of sexual function
    of the male: anafrodisia; satyriasis; priapism
    of the female: nymphomania; hysteria.

Pinel rejected the view that the neuroses proper were associated with anatomical lesions and put forward 'moral' or 'sympathetic' causes. He explained the former in terms of the classical doctrine of the 'passions' or 'affections of the soul' which he dressed up in contemporary garb;[188] the 'sympathetic reactions' Pinel described as resulting from 'sympathetic' influences from the stomach, organs of reproduction or other parts of the body affecting the brain at a distance. This view led directly to Broussais's doctrine of 'sympathetic neuroses'.

Influential writers not only affect the future but also their immediate contemporaries and as a direct result of Pinel's *Nosographie*, a number of nosologies were published during the early years of the nineteenth century. These books and the many editions and translation of the *Nosographie* made the concept of neurosis accessible to most European physicians. The ensuing uniformity of views imposed a new conceptual and terminological order which previous systems, such as Cullen's, were never able to achieve.

Amongst Pinel's followers, Anthelme Richerand deserves some attention, especially for the way in which he classified the neuroses in the fourth edition of his *Nosographie chirurgicale* (1815). In the first edition (1805) he just adapted the principles of vitalism to surgical pathology: in his first *class* he included 'lesions common to all organic systems' such as wounds, ulcers and osteoarthritic diseases (in the manner traditionally done by surgeons); he dealt with the conditions affecting individual organic systems in the remaining seven *classes*.[189]

Richerand modified this classification in the fourth edition of his book and, although still under the influence of vitalism, he took into consideration the anatomoclinical view; his intention was to develop a classification that was useful to surgical practice. He mentioned three classes:

  I Physical alterations
 II Organic or structural alterations
III Vital alterations.

In the first class he included surgical states such as solutions of continuity, morbid adhesions, separations, retentions and foreign bodies. In the second class are grouped scroffula, carcinoma, polyps, cysts and ossifications. The third class he subdivided into 'esthenia', 'asthenia', 'asphyxia' and 'ataxia': the 'esthenias' included essential fevers, inflammations and 'active haemorrhages'; the 'asthenias', ricketts, scurvy, caries, passive haemorrhages and 'nervous weakness'; gangrene and necrosis are considered as 'asphyxias' and the neuroses as 'ataxias'.[190]

'Physical lesion' is defined as 'the mechanical consequence of a cause acting mechanically';[191] 'organic lesion' as: 'severe and complete lesion leading to a loss of identity of the diseased tissue'.[192]

'Vital lesion' referred to 'impairment of the properties that distinguish the living body from inert matter, such as sense and contractility. Difficulty in teasing these two properties apart has led physiologists to bring them together under the common term 'vitality'.[193]

The nature of the relationship between 'organic' and 'vital alteration' is unclear in the work of Richerand: 'Some vital lesions are not associated with physical lesion or organic alteration. Thus in gout there is no observable alteration of the optic nerve nor can any lesion of the nervous system be identified in the vesanias and epilepsies... Vital lesions however may occasionally produce structural alterations; but even in these cases they should be considered as essentially different...'[194]

The 'ataxias' Richerand defined as states caused by alterations of the properties of life, and amongst them he included a number of 'diseases which the authors refer to as neurosis'.[195] The neuroses not classified as 'ataxias' he grouped as 'nervous weaknesses' hemeralopia, dyspepsia, anafrodisia and idiocy) together with the 'asthenias'. Richerand's definition of neurosis is similar to Cullen's: 'anomalies of sense and contractibility' and includes the neuralgias, the paroxysmal phenomena (tetanus, asthma, whooping cough, epilepsy etc.) and the vesanias; this latter group comprised mania, melancholia, dementia, hypochondria and 'the hysterical'.

While some followers of Pinel repeated the classification of the *Nosographie* others re-ordered its classes according to particular interpretations of Enlightenment medicine. Amongst the former feature J. J. Duret with his *Tableau* (1815) and J. L. Alibert whose *Nosologie naturelle* (1817–25) was the last important manifestation of *more botanico* taxonomy in French medicine; amongst the latter should be mentioned the systems of J. T. Tourdes (1802) and of E. Tourtelle (1799). Examples of both groups abound both inside and outside French medicine.[196]

The concept of neurosis during the first anatomoclinical period: Georget's revision

Pinel's view of the neuroses, although transitional and only partially anatomoclinical, was influential on their evolution in that it made them lose their character of 'general diseases'. In spite of this transformation, the neuroses proved resistant to anatomical reduction and remained as an island of functional pathology in the midst of the new morphological programme.

The new pathology soon abandoned its vitalistic principles and its emphasis on symptomatology and restricted itself to the anatomo-clinical approach. This change increased its incompatibility with the concept of neurosis and the ensuing impasse was considered by many to be unresolvable. The feeling of unease that has accompanied the concept of neuroses ever since dates back to this period. This conceptual change also created expectations amongst the reforming physicians of this period that the gradual discovery of specific lesions would lead to the disappearance of this nosological class and that the concept of neuroses was redundant.

This expectation was ninety per cent fulfilled. As pathological research advanced, most of the conditions then described as neuroses soon proved to have organic basis (or alternatively to be mere symptoms). On the other hand a number of putative lesions such as endometritis and oophoritis (assumed to cause hysteria) and gastric or hepatic lesions (assumed to cause hypochondria) were unable to stand scientific scrutiny.

The concept of neuroses therefore was considered as provisional and often as vague and unscientific. However authors such as Laennec still made use of it. In his *Traité de l'auscultation médiate* he wrote when dealing with the 'organic diseases' of the lungs: 'I shall now examine the diseases of this organ which are accompanied by no structural change and might result from disorder in its fluids or in that part that causes it to move; namely, and to utilize the modern language, the nervous disorders'.[197] Few authors during this period however felt able to play down the difficulties that the concept of neurosis posed to the new medicine.

It seemed clear that a drastic revision of the concept of neuroses was needed: such was undertaken by Etienne Jean Georget (1795–1828), a member of Esquirol's school, in his posthumously published entry to the twenty-one volume *Dictionnaire de Médecine* (1840).[198]

The relevance of this contribution can be illustrated by the fact that the concept of neurosis was kept in currency only by those writers who came directly or indirectly under his influence. This explains its persistence in French medicine and in the medicine of countries such as Germany, which after its romantic period had come under the aegis of the Paris school. On the other hand the term vanished in countries like Great Britain, which, in spite of having assimilated some of the principles of the Paris school, followed in the end an independent path.

In his entry of less than twenty pages Georget made three fundamental contributions:

1. A critique of early concepts of neurosis;
2. A defence of the need to retain the concept; and,
3. An adaptation of the term to the conceptual demands of anatomopathology.

First of all he challenged the views of those who wanted to discard the concept such as Pinel, Broussais and the anatomoclinicians. In relation to Pinel's views Georget wrote:

> Pinel could be criticized for not having tried hard enough to differentiate the neuroses from other diseases or for having accepted uncritically, as members of this group, conditions that have for long been known to be associated with organic lesions. For example, apoplexy is thus classified, in spite of the fact that Morgagni had already described its pathological changes... [199]

Georget considered Pinel as 'out of date' and his methodology and anatomoclinical view insufficient to deal with the problems of the new medicine.

In relation to Broussais, Georget took a different attitude: 'It must be iterated, Broussais has not been understood. The neuroses which he specifically mentions by name should be included amongst the inflammations. Other neuroses are referred to only in a general way and no facts are provided to back up his claims...'[200] Georget criticized the speculative view of Broussais who in the absence of evidence, considered the neuroses as lesional diseases; for Georget Broussais's view was 'unsupported by the facts'. He implicitly levelled the same accusation against Roche, 'a sensible member of the new school' whose views he critically summarized.[201]

Georget explored the clash between the concept of neurosis and the anatomoclinical view and followed up the individual fate of those neuroses that had been accepted by Pinel. Thus he found that the 'neuroses of the senses' can be reduced to being aberrations of disposition (myopia) or secondary to organic problems (amaurosis, deafness). Apoplexy he defined as a 'cluster of symptoms resulting from general congestion of the brain, from stagnation of the blood or from encephalic disorganization'; idiocy he put down to a congenital disorganization of the brain resulting from multiple causes; hydrophobia, tetanus, whooping cough etc. he retained as diseases associated with known lesions.[202]

Georget evaluated the various lesions claimed at the time to be related to those states he was to consider later as neuroses proper. For example, he quoted Martinet's view on the neuralgias as inflammatory conditions of the nerves; Rostan's view of asthma as a cardiac lesion and Laennec's alternative pulmonary theory; Pujol's view of hypochondria as hepatitis and of hysteria as chronic endometritis; Cazauvieilh and Bouchet's view of epilepsy as a chronic inflammation of the white matter; and, the view that certain forms of *folie* may result from 'phlegmasia encephalica'.[203] This systematic assessment of the way that the anatomoclinical method had been applied to the concept of neurosis led Georget to conclude that 'According to this view it would seem the neuroses do not exist'.[204]

This conclusion he rejected. He believed that, although about ninety per cent of the labours of the anatomoclinicians had borne fruit and many conditions could no longer be considered as neurosis, there was still a small group of morbid states that deserved such name:

> in my articles on *epilepsy*; *madness*; *gastralgia*; *hypochondria* and *hysteria* (in the Dictionnaire de Médecine) I have dealt with a number of conditions which must be differentiated both from the phlegmasias and the disorganizations. They exhibit their own characteristics and it is right that they be grouped under the terms neuroses or nervous diseases, which are anyway used to refer to these conditions.[205]

Then Georget offered a positive definition:

> The diseases which I shall refer to as neuroses are chronic, not dangerous, intermittent, without fever, able in appearance to occasion great suffering which often leads one to believe that something very serious is going on; and are accompanied by minor or no post-mortem evidence of organic damage. The neuroses include periodic headache;

madness, hypochondria, catalepsy, chorea, hysteria, asthma, nervous palpitations, gastralgia with or without vomiting and neuralgias.[206]
It is hardly surprising that Georget's revision was so influential. With the usual French clarity of exposition and analysis, he carried out an objective and self-critical appraisal and concluded that the anatomoclinical method was insufficient to deal with the neuroses. His general contribution, appearing in a prestigious medical dictionary was instrumental in the retention of the concept of neurosis in European medicine. His definition and list of specific neuroses, however, suffered a different fate and were soon to be superseded.

The anatomoclinical concept of neurosis from Georget to Charcot: 'functional localization'

The retention of the concept of neuroses during the anatomoclinical period was achieved at the price of forfeiting the double principle of anatomical lesion and localization and of continuing with mere symptomatological description. It is not surprising therefore that the subsequent evolution of the concept is marked by attempts to regain at least one of these principles. One such effort, aimed at a 'functional localization' of the neurosis, was initiated by Achille Louis Foville (1799–1878) who, like Georget, was a member of Esquirol's school and an important worker in neurophysiology.[207]

Foville's main contribution to the theory of neurosis is his article of 1834 in the *Dictionnaire de Médecine et de Chirurgie pratiques*.[208] His view was forceful: 'It seems to me that the fundamental question concerning the neuroses, which must be considered as conditions essentially physiological in nature, has not yet been understood; as a consequence, under this term a number of conditions of unknown cause have been grouped'.[209] Foville endeavoured to characterize the neuroses from the physiopathological viewpoint: 'Although we are all committed to identifying physical modifications, it is important to recourse to pathological physiology in order to clarify the problem of the neuroses... and thus solve the conundrum'.[210] This task he himself undertook within the orthodox framework of the anatomo-clinical view: 'to claim that the neuroses are diseases characterized by symptoms indicative of alterations of the nervous system which so far remain unidentified, is too narrow a view...I believe it is better to define the neuroses as diseases that, to judge by their symptoms, must be localized in the nervous system, but that show no observable alteration'.[211]

This view of Foville's gave rise to the so-called period of 'functional localization' in the history of the concept of neurosis. Foville attempted to identify experimentally a causal link between neurosis and the state of the blood vessels in the nervous system: 'All manifestations of vital activity, whether normal or not, depend upon the reciprocal activity of blood vessels and nerves'.[212] Anatomo-clinicians at the time adopted from Foville only the principle of localization but disregarded his physiopathological view. Thirty years later Brown-Séquard found his task of developing a similar physio-pathological view of the neurosis facilitated by the fact that by then the 'functional' had become a predominant concept.[213]

In the decade following the publication of Georget's and Foville's work (1840–1850) most anatomoclinical writers fully adopted the localizationist principle without, however, taking the argument to its final conclusions insofar as it applied to the neuroses. In opposition to this, works published after 1860 began to suggest specific localizations for the neuroses and no longer preoccupied themselves with their general aspects.

Typical texts from this period are the monograph by A. A. Tardieu: *Jusq'à quel point le diagnostique anatomique peut-il éclairer le traitement des névroses?* (1844) and the entry on 'Névroses' for the *Compendium de Médecine pratique* by Monneret and L. Fleury (1845). Both works accepted without hesitation the application of the principle of functional localization to the neuroses[214] which Tardieu defined as: 'episodic conditions without fever and localized somewhere in the nervous system, with tendency to spread and which are characterized by alteration of its functions but without identifiable lesion of solids or fluids'.[215] Monneret and Fleury, in turn, defined neurosis as 'apyrexial disease localized centrally or peripherally in the nervous system but without identifiable or primitive lesion'.[216]

Foville's physiopathological view is nowhere to be found in these works that treat the principle of localization as little more than theoretical aspiration. For example, the *Compendium* continues classifying the neuroses according to symptomatology.

However after 1860 the anatomoclinicians began to suggest specific localization for the neuroses showing clear disregard to their general aspects. Two books can be mentioned in this context: *Klinik der Nervenkrankheiten* (1870) by the Austrian Moritz Rosenthal and *Traité de Pathologie Interne* (1872) by the French Sigismond Jaccoud.[217]
The structure of Rosenthal's book illustrates well the point just made: he attempts to order not only the neurological diseases but also the neuroses in terms of their anatomical localization starting in the meninges and encephalus down to the peripheral nerves. However only in the case of 'the neurosis of the spinal cord' was he able to achieve his objective: together with myelitis and other spinal cord diseases he included the 'neuroses of the spinal cord' under which he classified the hyperaesthetic and depressive forms of 'spinal irritation'. This latter concept considered by Rosenthal only as a particular neurosis, will be dealt with later on.[218]
The remaining neuroses posed more difficulty. Under two categories: 'spinal and cerebral neuroses accompanied by cramp' and 'neuroses accompanied by tremor and inco-ordination' Rosenthal included epilepsy, eclampsia, catalepsia, tetanus, hydrophobia, paralysis agitans, the choreas etc.... He created another category for the 'neuroses of the sexual organs' which comprised seminal loss, impotence, aespermatosis etc.... Equally unsatisfactory was the localization of the 'trophic and vasomotor neuroses' which he conjured up by invoking the physiopathological view and focusing on those conditions which were supposed to be associated with the autonomic nervous system. Similar problems arose regarding the 'toxic neuroses and nervous disorders associated with febrile conditions, anaemic and reflex paralyses' in relation to which Rosenthal once again abandoned the localizationist principle and resorted to an aetiological criterion. Hysteria also presented him with difficulties: 'In addition to the diseases of brain and spinal cord just mentioned, hysteria and its various forms will now be dealt with as it can also give rise to the symptoms already described'.[219] But when referring to the assumed pathological anatomy of this disorder all that Rosenthal could do was dismiss the uterine pathology hypothesis and put his faith in the progress of science.[220] In his effort to offer at least a modicum of localization he resorted to the hypothesis of 'spinal irritation': 'irritation...can start in the spinal cord, spread up to the

brain stem and generate more or less severe alteration of cerebral activity...'[221]

Rosenthal included in his work an adequate inventory of known anatomical lesions and avoided dealing with all general issues by directly placing the neuroses, together with the other nervous diseases, within his anatomical programme. Thus, his work stepped beyond the wishful thinking of Monneret and Fleury or Tardieu by actually attempting to localize the neuroses, albeit in a physiological way. Sadly the results were meagre for 'spinal irritation' (which in any case was conceptually possible only in the context of the physiopathological view) was the only condition in which the localizationist principle could be fulfilled. The remaining neuroses could only achieve vague localizations and, in the case of hysteria, not even this was possible.

Jaccoud dealt with the neuroses in the first volume of his *Traité de Pathologie interne* after having studied the diseases of the brain, spinal cord, autonomic nervous system and peripheral nerves. He developed a 'clear and distinct' classification based on the localizationist principle:

1. Brain neuroses (Mental diseases)
2. Cerebrospinal neuroses (epilepsy, hysteria, catalepsy)
3. Brainstem neuroses (paralysis agitans, chorea, tetanus)
4. Peripheral neuroses (neuralgias, anaesthesias, hyperkinesias, akinesias)

Even more interesting is Jaccoud's view of the neuroses:

The (nervous) diseases just described are recognized specifically by their symptoms, which suggest localization in the nervous system, and named in terms of the constant lesions which accompany them; they exhibit therefore a symptomatic or physiological aspect (that relates to localization) and an anatomical aspect (that relates to nature). On the other hand the diseases to be described presently under the generic name of neuroses only exhibit the former characteristic, namely, localization which is based on a physiological analysis of the symptoms; the anatomical criterion cannot yet be fulfilled and therefore the question of their nature remains uncertain.

Although postmortem examinations may frequently show lesions which in principle can be considered as sufficient to develop a pathogenic view of some neuroses, their inconsistent appearance undermines their value. This point, I believe to be important namely that even if lesions are identified in relation to each disease, unless these show a consistent pattern, the situation will be no better than it is now; what is needed is the unequivocal and persistent identification of lesions in relation to each neurosis, such as, for example, haemorrhage and cerebral sclerosis which are always present in the diseases that carry the same name'.[222]

This clear account illustrates well the confrontation of the anatomoclinical view with the concept of neuroses and requires no further comment. It also gives substance to the hypothesis put forward in this book, that the concept of neurosis constituted a formidable stumbling block for the development of a new pathology based on the anatomoclinical method. Although the elimination of the concept seemed feasible during the early stages it soon became clear that this premature hope had been based on the facile acceptance of views which were only superficially 'objective' or 'scientific' and which would not stand rigorous scientific scrutiny; for example, such procedure rendered the uterine theory of hysteria untenable.

At any rate the well-advertised disappearance of the neuroses only referred to about ninety per cent of the group. The fate of the remaining ten per cent, for which no characteristic lesion had been identified, was entrusted to the future and to the advance of science. But this procrastinatory solution, shared by a number of psychiatrists in our own century, was unsatisfactory to those who had gone deeply into the problem of the neuroses for they believed that mere reduction in numbers was less important than dealing with that irreducible core for which pathological explanation had not yet been found.

Confronted by this difficulty, the anatomoclinical view tried harder. In the event what resulted was a questioning of foundations and a search for conceptual limits of the kind well illustrated by Jaccoud's quotation. Medicine is never more self-conscious of its theoretical basis than when it is faced with some irreducible facts. In accordance with this strategy, anatomoclinical medicine dismissed all easy answers and squarely confronted the crucial issue: since anatomical localization was not to be achieved, functional localization had to be accepted as the way out of the labyrinth.

Around the period during which Rosenthal and Jaccoud were publishing their work, J. M. Charcot had started his and the anatomoclinical view found in his writings both its crowning moment and its dénouement. The master of La Salpêtrière concentrated his efforts on hysteria, the *grande névrose*, for this condition posed the problem of the neuroses at its sharpest. He transformed the 'functional localization' view, which he had inherited, into the 'transitory lesion' principle and collated the results of more than half a century of research by French anatomoclinicians.

During the early decades of the century two interpretative theories of hysteria had vied for supremacy: the 'uterine neurosis' view[223] sponsored by Louyer-Villermay (1816) and E. F. Dubois (1837), and the 'encephalopathy' view[224], represented by Georget (1821) and Voisin (1826). These localizationist doctrines were criticized by P. Briquet in his important '*Traité clinique et thérapeutique de l'hystérie*' (1859)[225], considered by Charcot and his followers as a seminal influence. Two aspects of this work are relevant to the doctrine developed at La Salpêtrière. Firstly there was Briquet's criticism of the accepted view of hysteria as always showing 'protean' symptomatology and his belief that this had to be studied empirically. The outcome of this work was the description of 'clear and distinct' boundaries for the 'convulsive hysteria' and the identification of its 'free intervals'; Briquet also described various clinical forms of catalepsy, sleepwalking and of 'hysterical equivalents' which were not accompanied by convulsions. Briquet's work was an important source for the ambitious nosological classification that Charcot was to undertake. The second influential aspect of Briquet's work was his dismissal of 'encephalopathy' as a cause of hysteria which he instead considered as 'a consequence of damage to that part of the brain that receives affective impressions';[226] he concluded that since this alteration soon finds expression in all the organism, hysteria must be a *maladie générale*. In the midst of a medical world bent on localizationism hysteria, the most representative of all neuroses, was thereby on the verge of regaining one of its original characteristics.

4: *The physiopathological view and the concept of neurosis*

The physiopathological view, the other dominant trend in nineteenth-century scientificonatural medicine, developed as a modification of the anatomoclinical view which must be considered as the very foundation of the new medicine. Its novelty was to emphasize the 'functional', which had been neglected by the great French writers and their followers, and to study objectively clinical and pathological dysfunctions. Laín Entralgo[227] has carried out a masterly study of the group of German authors (Wunderlich, Griesinger, Frerichs and Traube) who occupied themselves with the notion of dysfunction. They presided over the modification of the anatomoclinical view under the influence of dynamic and idealist views received from an earlier period of German medicine. The dynamic processes of old, rid of all speculative elements, adapted themselves to the new view: *Naturphilosophie* became *Naturwissenschaft*.

The preponderance of the German school should not conceal the fact that the French and the British also sponsored the physiopathological view. In the Paris of the early nineteenth century the only view that kept the notion of the 'functional' alive was the 'heterodox' doctrine of Broussais. The so-called 'Physiological medicine', although occasionally exaggerated, showed a commendable insistence on physiopathology.[228] Its early demise did not prevent '*Médecine physiologique*' from influencing both the orthodox French anatomoclinical view and the British physiopathological school. However the main origin of the latter must still be sought in the influential views of John Hunter who interested himself both in the experimental analysis of function and in its post-mortem concomitants.[229]

The failure of anatomoclinical medicine to redefine the neuroses in morphological and localizationist terms encouraged the early

59

application of the physiopathological view. This attempted to provide a positive definition of the neuroses which replaced the old morphologically negative definition. The ensuing development was expressed in a number of ways; these will be explored under six headings:

The 'physiological medicine' of Broussais

The disappearance of the term *neurosis* in British medicine

The concept of 'spinal irritation'

The reflex functional nervous diseases

The so-called 'trophic and vasomotor neuroses'

Broussais's 'médecine physiologique'

François Joseph Victor Broussais (1772–1838)[230] has been cast by medical historians in the invidious role of antagonist of the great Laennec; also well known are his speculations on the doctrine of 'irritation' and on 'gastroenteritis' which led to catastrophic therapeutic measures such as the weakening diet and bleeding. Broussais believed that life is maintained in the organism by the 'irritation' produced in the respiratory and digestive systems by external stimuli. Health would consist in moderate 'irritation' and hence pathological excess or want of irritation would lead to 'irritative' and 'esthenic' disease, respectively. For this belief three sources can be identified: the speculative system of John Browns's, Bichat's idea of life, and pathological anatomy. Broussais adopted the principle of local lesions but his hasty disposition led him to speculate that an inflammation of the digestive tract, a 'gastroenteritis' was the primary anatomical alteration of all 'general diseases'. The causal chain he postulated was simple: abnormal 'irritation' in the digestive tract leads to inflammation which spreads to the nervous system and gives rise to all manner of symptoms.

It would be unfair, however, to neglect the positive aspects of Broussais's work such as his incisive attack on nosological ontologism and on the concept of fever as an 'essential disease'. Equally important is his insistence, during a period when all efforts went into morphology, on the important role that physiology must play in pathological explanation. His contribution to the evolution of the concept of neurosis can be said to stem from this keenness on the 'functional'.

His views on this topic must be understood against the context of
his general belief in the phenomenon of nervous 'sympathy':
  The nerves are the only means of transmission of irritation
  thus providing the organic bases for the sympathies. Morbid
  sympathies are mediated by the same mechanism that
  operates during the state of health; the only difference being
  that in the morbid case the nerves convey an excess of
  irritation which violates the laws of life... Morbid sympathies
  that manifest themselves in organic phenomena are called
  organic sympathies; those which manifest themselves in
  pain, muscle contraction, voluntary contraction and mental
  aberration...are called relational sympathies... Irritation
  leads to accumulation of blood in tissues and the ensuing
  swelling, redness and heat may disorganize the irritated part,
  resulting in inflammation... Inflammation may give origin
  to relational sympathies which some authors have tended to
  consider as the predominant phenomena; to these the name
  of *neurosis* has been given.[231]
These quotations from the *Propositions* summarize Broussais's
views well. Neuroses are but observational artefacts created by
diseases exhibiting a predominance of 'morbid sympathies'. Broussais
subscribed to a heterodox form of the anatomoclinical view and this
led him to achieve, albeit speculatively, what had been the objective
all along of this view in relation to the neuroses, namely, to reduce
these conditions to simple theoretical entities and to explain their
clinical manifestations in terms of an anatomical lesion. While
orthodox anatomoclinicians tried to reach this objective by searching
for specific lesions and hence eroding the concept piecemeal, Broussais
attempted this at one fell swoop by declaring 'gastroenteritis' to be
the origin of all neurotic processes. He suggested a functional
hypothesis according to which all neurotic phenomena find their
pathogenesis in the 'morbid sympathies' conveyed by the nervous
system.
  But the anatomoclinical climate reigning in France at the time did
not allow this physiopathological view to thrive. Broussais's speculative functionalism continued into the next historical period but
without the imaginative fancies that characterized Broussais's work

it was less fruitful. It will be seen below how this functional view encouraged Roche (an author occupying a transitional position between Broussism and the orthodox anatomoclinical view) to postulate that the neuroses were diseases with 'imperceptible' anatomical lesions and also led Foville (who approached physiopathology from the vantage point of anatomoclinical medicine) to put forward the hypothesis of 'functional localization', relevant to the history of the neuroses. Although the dynamic view held by the two French authors remained under the control of their morphological thought, it also contained seeds of physiological thinking which were later to germinate.

The attractive and unfortunate Louis Charles Roche (1790–1875)[232] is mainly remembered as the co-author (with the surgeon Sanson) of a pathology treatise very popular in a number of European countries. He is not usually considered as a follower of Broussais, although as a young man he vigorously defended the 'Médecine physiologique'. In later years he gravitated towards the official anatomoclinical view and in his mature work he chose a via media. The doctrine of 'irritation' is still important to his work and his view on the neurosis stems from it.

Roche endeavoured to develop an anatomoclinical nosology and a classification. He considered the 'material alterations that take place in tissues and fluids' as the 'real basis for classification'.[233] The thirteen types of 'alterations of solids' he listed are mostly anatomopathological in character: 'gangrene', 'disorganizations', 'morbid products' etc... Two of these however betray his Broussism: 'irritations' and 'asthenias'; the former 'consisting in a reduced flow of the fluids that irrigate the tissues, leading to an increase in irritability'.[234] Amongst the six types of 'irritation', together with the inflammatory and haemorrhagic conditions, Roche placed the 'nervous irritation or neurosis'. On this he wrote

> irritation not always increases flux in the affected tissues
> and then pain and disorder of function may be the only
> signs present. This particular type of irritation we have
> called *nervous irritation* or *neurosis* and defined as augmented
> organic activity in a given tissue without fluid increase. In
> the same way in which the praeternatural congestion of
> blood in a tissue constitutes the pathognomonic feature of

inflammation, accumulation of nervous fluid constitutes the fundamental character of the neuroses.[235]

Roche's model is simple and requires no explanation. Working within the confines of a system based on the principle of the anatomical lesion he was able to make room for the functional view, taken from Broussais's speculative work and, on this basis, postulate the notion of 'imperceptible lesion' as the foundation of the neurosis: 'The accumulation of nervous fluid is as material a phenomenon as the congestion of blood in inflamed tissue. The only difference resides in the fact...that the nervous fluid (like electric fluid) is not visible; the similarity between the two is becoming increasingly clearer.'[236]

Roche defined asthenia, which he did not regard as a neurosis, as resulting from a 'lesser flow of fluid than in the natural state, resulting in a reduction in irritability',[237] that is, as opposite to 'nervous irritation'.

The disappearance of the term 'neurosis' from British medicine

British physicians had led the field in pathological anatomy during the late eighteenth century. Together with their colleagues in Europe they soon incorporated the French contributions and many in the Edinburgh, Dublin and London Hospitals began to sponsor the new medicine. The view they developed, markedly different from the one held by their continental contemporaries, owed a great deal to the thought of John Hunter, the great surgeon of the Enlightenment. Hunter agreed with the Paris school on the need to link up clinical observation with post-mortem data but put greater emphasis on the experimental analysis of function. Apart from the Hunterian views German physiopathological medicine was also influential around the mid-nineteenth century on British thinking particularly on the Edinburgh school. The strong presence of the physiopathological view amongst British physicians explains why, unlike their French counterparts, anatomoclinicians in Great Britain were from early times aware of functional concepts.[238]

As in France, and due to similar historical reasons, the concept of neurosis became unpopular in Great Britain. But while its persistent use in France was guaranteed by the rehabilitatory and analytic work of no less a man than Georget, nothing of the kind occurred in Great Britain. Consequently the term was to vanish, for over half a century, from the medical writings of the very country that had coined it in the first place.[239]

But the clinical and pathological phenomena to which the word neurosis referred, continued being debated under different names, such as 'Spinal irritation' or 'Reflex functional nervous diseases', which were but explanatory images created by British physiopathology.

The concept of 'spinal irritation'

Benjamin Travers, one of the best surgeons from Astley Cooper's school at Guy's Hospital, suggested in 1824 the term 'constitutional irritation' to name a general pathogenic mechanism, mediated by the nervous system, on the basis of which it was possible to explain how generalized effects could follow minimal local alterations.[240] Ten years later he broadened the concept to account for the mechanisms involved in other nervous conditions.[241]

The sources of Travers's ideas were the work of Broussais,[242] the neurophysiological discoveries of Charles Bell and his own surgical experience which helped him to temper the Broussonian influence. The real interest of Travers and Cooper was to identify the mechanisms that explained why intense general effects could follow insignificant local lesions. Small wonder, therefore, that they adopted Broussais's concept of 'irritation' which they understood as a fundamental pathological process similar to inflammation but unaccompanied by hyperaemia or exudate. Available neurophysiological knowledge provided Travers and Cooper with a ready-made mechanism to explain how irritation could spread to any region of the organism; for example they felt able to account in 'physiological terms' for the systemic effect of erysipelar infections originating in small wounds. This early British version, conceptualized 'irritation' in the simplest of manners, as 'of local origin', 'constitutional' and having general repercussion, and proceeded to apply it to all clinical problems that were considered as 'general manifestations of a local process'. Astley Cooper applied this hypothesis in his *Lectures on Surgery* to clinical situations as diverse as traumatic shock following a fracture, the systemic effect of dental abscesses and the 'general maladie' that might follow bites.[243]

The obvious crudeness of this hypothesis reduced its influence and apart from Travers and Cooper only Benjamin C. Brodie[244] is known to have subscribed to it in its unmodified version. Modified versions however abounded, for example C. J. B. Williams and J. Crawford emphasized the 'fundamental' character of 'irritation' which they considered to be the initial stage of inflammation[245]; in this regard Travers himself had already thought of the possibility that 'irritation' might after all be followed by secondary lesions. Other authors attempted to take advantage of the pathogenic hypothesis contained in the notion of irritation and playing by the anatomoclinical rules of the time sought for it an anatomical localization. Thus Charles Bell and the well-known John Abercrombie[246] localized 'irritation' in the spinal cord.

Yet another view must also be discussed in this context. Player[247] published a monograph in 1821 suggesting that some of the neuralgias and neuroses resulted from pressure exercised on the cord by the cervical vertebrae processes; he left however the nature of the relevant spinal cord changes unclear and his notion of '*spinal disease*' remained vague although well distinguished from inflammation. The very title of Player's influential book *Irritation of the Spinal Nerves* betrays its kinship with Travers's ideas although it can be said that its central point was original and independent. C. Brown published in 1828[248] a book of the same title *Irritation of the Spinal Nerves* but his hypothesis, intended to explain certain 'neuropathic states', is contrived and alien to the then prevalent view of 'irritation' as a general pathological process. In Brown's peculiar notion, irritation results from compression on the spinal nerves caused by slight vertebral displacements, themselves produced by spasmodic contraction of the spinal muscles.

The blending of these two points of view, the pathological and the clinical, was undertaken during the following years by a number of authors who attempted to explain neuralgic and neurotic conditions by means of 'nervous irritation'. But as this notion became circumscribed to the spinal cord the associated explanation also became circumscribed to 'spinal irritation'.

Darwal[249] suggested in 1829 that spinal and cerebral irritation may cause 'generalized neuralgias' and some of these he equated, as the French Valleix was to do later, with the neuroses. He also believed that in these cases there was no nervous lesion present and that the functional alteration resulted from centrally induced hyperaemia or circulatory 'irritation'. This view was adopted almost unchanged in 1829 by the great French neurologist Ollivier (d'Angers)[250] and was reformulated in Britain by Teale[251] who considered 'spinal irritation' as tantamount to generalized neuralgia and believed that tenderness on apophysiary spots (Player's sign) eventually developed in all chronic nervous diseases.

Tate[252] in his *Treatise on Hysteria* (1830) also considered the tender spots as relevant to the diagnosis of hysteria and suggested that irritation of the spinal cord could cause all hysterical manifestations. However, the primary origin of irritation was for him still the uterus, thereby subscribing to the 'uterine theory'. Tate bridged the gap between the *grande névrose* of Charcot and the vague neuralgic and neurotic ailments of Darwal and Teale. His views illustrate well the many explanatory tasks to which was put the notion of 'spinal irritation'.

During the following years many sponsored the view that *most nervous diseases* were characterized by tender spots on the spine and resulted from non-inflammatory spinal cord dysfunctions without anatomical change. Amongst these workers the American Isaac Parrish[253] must be mentioned; his efforts to popularize the term 'spinal irritation' led the German Baas[254], years later, to believe that he had been its creator. The British Turnbull[255] also belongs in this group.

William and Daniel Griffin (1834) attempted a more precise localization of irritation in the spinal cord and considered intermittent fever to be a form of 'spinal irritation'[256] thereby widening this pathogenic hypothesis. The fact that during this period it is still possible to find writers subscribing to the nervous origin of fever, confirms the influence of Cullen's 'neuralpathology'. The expansion of the concept of 'spinal irritation' during this period was such that it engulfed clinical conditions that thirty years before had been classified as neuroses; even intermittent fever came to be considered as a vasomotor neurosis.

The highest point in the evolution of the concept of 'spinal irritation' however was reached not in Great Britain but in Germany where the new pathogenic theory was soon adopted by eminent physicians such as Stilling, Türck and Canstatt.[257] It was however the work of Enz[258] that legitimized the use of irritation as a pathogenic mechanism applicable to all nervous diseases. In keeping with the speculative trends of the transitional period to which he belonged, Enz widened the boundaries of the concept of 'spinal irritation' to include, not only all nervous diseases, but also intermittent fever, dyspepsia, cough, hemoptysis, vomiting and all manner of colics. Roux[259] was right to consider Enz's view as a monistic explanation similar to Broussais's 'gastroenteritis'.

Enz's overemphasis was severely criticized. The work of Aaron Mayer[260] (1849) must be mentioned in this respect as it put out of fashion (*Modetheorie*) the concept of 'spinal irritation' in German medicine. The great neurologist E. Von Leyden[261] dismissed the notion of spinal irritation which he considered as a mere name for a symptom and S. Key went as far as including it amongst the symptoms of hysteria. Niemeyer and d'Imman also disregarded the concept and limited themselves to explaining the tender spots as a simple myalgia.[262]

'Spinal irritation' lost its pathogenic role before the middle of the nineteenth century. However, it continued featuring, although with a different meaning, in the medical literature. This was the period during which French authors began to consider 'spinal irritation' as a specific form of neurosis.

Even before its popularity had waned French authors had already reduced its area of competence. For example, Olliver (d'Angers)[263] in his monograph of 1837 referred to spinal irritation as a mere nosological entity, in spite of the fact that he still subscribed to Darwall's view on spinal hyperaemia.

Valleix, Monneret and Fleury[264] regarded 'spinal irritation' and dorsal intercostal neuralgia as one and the same condition. Far more popularity was reached, however, by Fonssagrive's[265] view that 'spinal irritation' and 'general neuralgia' were equivalent; this latter condition had been described by Valleix and his disciple Leclerc.[266]

Twenty years after Fonssagrive's work, Armaingaud reiterated that: 'the concept of spinal irritation means *more* than neuralgia but it also means *less* than general neurosis with which it has been identified...'[267]

'Spinal irritation' occupied, after its transformation into a specific neurosis, an intermediate position between hysteria and the neuralgias. As an 'intermediate neurosis' it is therefore found in all the books published during this period: Erichsen, Hammond, Axenfeld, Rosenthal and Erb.[268] This mid-region was already well populated by a number of 'intermediate' neuroses and with these 'spinal irritation' was in due course compared. These intermediate neuroses will be explored later on together with the new concept of 'neurasthenia' or 'asthenic spinal irritation', which was the last fruit of the changeable concept of 'spinal irritation' and which was to cannibalize the entire group of 'intermediate neuroses'.

The 'reflex functional nervous diseases'

Physiopathological medicine also made use of the reflex mechanism to explain paralyses and other functional nervous disorders. The first well-developed formulation of the reflex doctrine can be found in the work of the British physician Whytt and the German Prochaska.[269]

Whytt had preceded Cullen in the Edinburgh Chair and been one of the main sponsors of the concept of 'nervous disease'[270]; he described well the 'nervous disorders' that resulted from visceral disease[271] which he (and some of his contemporaries) called 'sympathetic', based on the belief that the underlying mechanism was an 'organic sympathy' mediated by the nervous system.

This speculative doctrine revived during the early nineteenth century, in spite of the conceptual changes that charaterized this period, thanks to the opportune availability of the reflex doctrine. Marshall Hall (1790–1857)[272] based this theory on experiments that demonstrated that destruction of the spinal grey matter abolished strychnine-induced contractions and which led him to suggest that reflex action was localized in the spinal cord. His interpretation however, was somewhat obscured by the added notion that there was a third excito-motor ('diastaltic') pathway. Hall distinguished between clinical disorders resulting from direct damage to the spinal cord and those caused reflexly by organic lesion sited elsewhere. In his book *On the diseases and derangements of the Nervous System* (1841) he made use of the reflex action to explain a gamut of clinical conditions from infantile paralysis, which he related to *dental irritation*[273], to spastic and paralytic states, tetanus, asthma, epilepsy and hysteria.[274] Echoes of Broussais are detected in the chapter on *Intestinal irritation* where Hall utilized this notion to explain reflex disorders. Also relevant to this theme is his *Aperçu du système spinal ou de la série des actions réflexes dans leurs applications à la pathologie et spécialement à l'épilepsie,*[275] which included papers he submitted to the *Académie des Sciences* in Paris.

Hall should be considered as the starting point of a prolonged historical process. The notion of 'reflex functional nervous disorder' became far clearer and better known at the hands of writers such as Stanley and Graves who, in spite of their feud over priority, provided this clinical category with adequate clinical content. For example, Stanley[276] reported cases of paraplegia showing a normal spinal cord but positive findings in the kidneys to support his view of paralysis as a reflex condition; Stanley did not generalize from his findings but *in passim* he mentioned that functional paralysis may also be associated with uterine pathology.

A broader generalization, based on a large clinical series, was offered by Graves, the Irish physician, in his *Clinical Lectures,*[277] perhaps the most popular textbook of clinical medicine in Europe during the first half of the nineteenth century. The cases reported by Graves relate mainly to intestinal inflammations and to peripheral disorders, a *frigore*. This book helped to spread the concept of reflex in the Continent; and Jaccoud's translation into French was widely read in Europe.[278] Graves's work was also taken as a model by the French movement of so-called 'pure clinicians' led by Trousseau.

The reflex doctrine merited also full treatment by the German physiopathological school, as the notion of 'spinal irritation' had done before. Henoch was one of the first to deal with the reflex functional nervous disorders and in 1845 published a monograph comparing motor disorders in man and in some domestic animals.[279] Romberg also adopted Graves's doctrine in the first edition of his neurological treatise[280] and distinguished three types of paralysis (and other nervous disorders), mediated by reflex mechanisms: (1) intestinal; (2) renal; and (3) uterine.

Its very simplicity gained the doctrine popularity but led to a proliferation of therapeutic methods. A number of surgical operations to treat 'nervous disorders' were suggested and performed during this period and as the doctrine reached its highest point during the 1840s even nephrectomy was considered as a valid indication in the treatment of paralysis and other reflex disorders of renal origin. This view managed to survive well into the twentieth century and in spite of criticism was used to justify hysterectomies and the removal of healthy teeth as treatments for certain neurological conditions.

The abuse of surgical procedures during the 1840s made physicians grow suspicious of the physiological foundations of the reflex theory which were soon found wanting. During the decade of the 1850s, many authors preferred to dissociate themselves from the theory, for example Romberg, in the third edition of this Treatise, called into question the evidential foundations of the reflex theory and proceeded to reclassify a number of disorders that in earlier editions he had related to reflex mechanism: disorders purportedly of uterine origin he placed with the nervous disorders of hysteria; disorders of putative intestinal origin he now explained as resulting from infection.[281]

These recantations however did not occasion the death of the theory. It remained both in medical practice and in medical ideology in at least three forms: (1) its original simple version; (2) in an anatomoclinical version, buttressed by descriptions of positive lesions; and (3) reformulated in terms of experimental physiopathology. The three versions found sponsors during the period 1860–1875, just before Charcot and Bernheim began to transform the concept of neurosis.

The 1864 monograph and the prestigious medical treatise[282] of the French physician Jaccoud illustrate well the first version. He adopted in both works a simple view of the reflex theory in spite of strong criticisms and explained functional paralysis as spinal cord fatigue caused by irritation; the latter he related to uterine, intestinal or bladder inflammation. But Jaccoud did not bother much to seek physiological data in support of his doctrine and, on close scrutiny his view is just a rehash of the old notions of 'irritation' and 'organic sympathy' inherited from eighteenth-century vitalism and well represented by Broussais during the nineteenth century.

The 'anatomoclinical' version was adopted by the British physician William W. Gull from Guy's Hospital in works published in 1856 and 1861. He called into question the assumption that no impairment of the spinal cord could be found, stating that microscopic lesions may be present in cases exhibiting no apparent lesion to the naked eye. For example he reported that the so-called 'urinary paraplegias' resulted from spinal cord involvement caused by bladder inflammation.[283] Robert Remak, the great German pathologist and microscopist concurred with this view and in his paper of 1860 he also reported that disorders of so-called spinal origin resulted from inflammation of the peripheral nerves.[284]

Ernst von Leyden, Professor of Clinical Medicine at Berlin and a renowned neurologist[285] was the most influential representative of the anatomoclinical version. In the 1865 paper on 'urinary paraplegias',[286] he reported two cases of bladder pathology involving the spinal cord and in his 1870 monograph on reflex paralysis he supported Remak's view.[287] In his classical Treatise on the diseases of the spinal cord (1874–1876) he wrote: 'Diseases of the bladder are not the only ones to involve the spinal cord, although not all do so by the same mechanism. Uterine and intestinal diseases also give rise to paraplegias...in these cases I have endeavoured to show that there is a transmission of neuritic inflammation to the spinal cord'.[288]

The physiopathological reformulation was conceptually superior to both the simple and the anatomoclinical versions of the doctrine. A model of this kind however required adequate experimental backing and this was provided by Charles Edouard Brown-Séquard, a bridging figure between British and French medicine.[289] His version of the doctrine was strict and based on his own experimental work; he had shown for example that stimulation of a peripheral nerve may trigger vasoconstriction in the spinal cord. In his book *Lectures on the Diagnosis and Treatment of Functional Nervous Affections* (1868) and in other works on vasomotor nerves and morbid and normal reflex action[290] Brown-Séquard developed the hypothesis that functional nervous disease was caused by a reduction in the activity of the spinal cord centres; the functional decline he explained as resulting from insufficient blood supply consequential upon irritation elsewhere in the body. Foville's old view of a putative link between circulation and nervous function was updated and given experimental support by Brown-Séquard. Most of all he showed that the reflexological view of the neurosis can survive provided that it is episodically reformulated and updated in terms of the facts of experimentation.

From 'intermediate neuroses' to neurasthenia

The concept of neurosis comprised from its very inception two groups of disorders: the 'major neuroses', namely hysteria and hypochondria, and the 'minor neuroses', that included the neuralgias, that is, the nineteenth century equivalent of the eighteenth century category *'dolores'*. Between 1850 and 1880 the two groups underwent important changes: the category 'major neurosis' became an exclusive name for hysteria; hypochondria broke up and its fragments were distributed out amongst different psychiatric diagnoses; and the neuralgias ceased to be considered as neuroses and were redefined as a separate group. The details of the historical process that led to these transformations will not be dealt with now; instead the gradual appearance of a number of intermediate neuroses which came to be placed between hysteria and the 'minor neuroses' will be described. One of these, named 'General Neuralgia' by Valleix in his 1841 Treatise on neuralgias,[291] developed as a result of his rejection of the view that the neuralgias *sensu stricto* were ever localized. But Valleix's contribution to the creation of the group of intermediate neuroses is not fundamental. In fact the development of the new category 'protean neuroses' only became possible after three changes had taken place: first, the conversion to the status of specific neuroses (the so-called 'spinal neuroses') of both 'spinal irritation' and the 'reflex doctrine', the two hypotheses once put forward as the common explanation for all functional nervous affections (including hysteria).

Secondly, the reflex explanatory mechanism which until then had been applicable only to the periphery was broadened to cover all parts of the central nervous system. Thus Brown-Séquard's vasomotor hypothesis was expanded in 1872 by the French physician Krishaber to cover also the 'cerebrocardiac neurosis'[292]; about the same time Leven (1879) redescribed in the same vein 'gastralgia' as a 'cerebrogastric neurosis'.[293]

Thirdly, 'spinal irritation' was subdivided into the 'esthenic' and 'asthenic' forms, corresponding to hyperfunction and hypofunction of the spinal cord, respectively. This classification, reminiscent of the views of Brown and Broussais, brought the concept of 'asthenia' to the forefront. It was defined as a state of spinal nervous exhaustion caused by the excessive 'irritation' that followed overstimulation. The early term 'asthenic spinal irritation' was eventually replaced by the shorter and more telling 'spinal neurasthenia'. The American physician Beard did for this condition what Krishaber and Leven had done for other ones, namely, extended the explanatory mechanism from the spinal cord to the cerebrum. In his 1868 and 1869 publications – which passed mostly unnoticed – Beard already had referred to 'cerebral exhaustion' as a process analogous to 'spinal exhaustion'. Likewise in the Anglo-Saxon world it became common to consider 'cerebral neurasthenia' and 'spinal neurasthenia' side by side.[294] The term *neurasthenia* (incidentally not coined by Beard) was already in use at the beginning of the nineteenth century in association with the doctrine of Brown and can be found in the medical dictionaries by Kraus (1831)[295] and Most (1836–1837).[296] These works belong to the German romantic period in which *Erregungstheorie* and other versions of Brownism were very influential. They define *neurasthenia* as a synonym of 'nervous weakness' and *neuroesthenia*, its opposite, as an equivalent of erethism.

Beard[297] believed 'neurasthenia' to be a functional disease of the brain occasioned by exhaustion resulting from intellectual overwork or tension, and which affected mainly professional and intellectual American men between the ages of sixteen and fifty (the years of sexual activity). Amongst the predisposing causes he mentioned dyspepsia; disorders of cerebral blood supply related to cardiovascular disease; sexual abuse; heredity; and climate. The symptomatology described by Beard is reminiscent of the clinical picture of 'spinal irritation' and includes both secondary symptoms and a pathognomonic feature consisting of a diffuse aching of the scalp considered as analogous[298] to the tender spine of 'spinal neurasthenia'.

From these humble origins neurasthenia was called upon to greater things and the conceptual readiness and social climate of the time made an immediate success of Beard's book published in 1880.[299] A year later the American physician Weir Mitchell[300] described the female form of neurasthenia and suggested a therapeutic programme. The successful adoption of the concept in many countries soon made people forget that it had been created to describe a disease in a particular country. Huchard (1883) was the first in France to introduce the concept of neurasthenia in the revised edition of Axenfeld's famous *Treatise on the neurosis*.[301] In Germany it was Ziemssen's monograph (1887)[302] that contributed (together with other works) to the diffusion of the concept.

But the decisive period in the evolution of neurasthenia is represented by the writing of Charcot and his group.[303] In his *Leçons du Mardi* (1888–1889)[304] the great man of the Salpêtrière included the concept into his classification of the neuroses and compared Beard's description with his own clinical observations of headache sufferers who also complained of aching and sensation of pressure on the scalp and whom he had called *Galeati*. Charcot then proceeded to reclassify them under Beard's category and, following his own analytic method, attempted to identify the stigmata and clinical types of neurasthenia as he had done for hysteria before. He compared both forms of neuroses and went as far as suggesting the existence of a hybrid form, hysteroneurasthenia that resulted from psychical trauma.

Charcot legitimized neurasthenia as a major neurosis, comparable only to hysteria, *la grande névrose* and his disciples, L. Bouveret (1890), F. Levillain (1891) and A. Mathieu (1892)[305] wrote monographs on the subject. This consecration of the neurasthenia concept had two main consequences: firstly, all 'protean' or intermediate neuroses were engulfed by neurasthenia; for example Bouchut's[306] 'nervousness' was considered as equivalent to neurasthenia and intermediate states such as 'asthenic spinal irritation' and the 'cerebrocardiac and cerebrogastric' neuroses became its partial manifestations. This phenomenon of assimilation determined that, of all the forms of neuroses created during the complex evolution of the concept, only hysteria and neurasthenia survived into the twentieth century. These two categories were to pose the central problem during the so-called psychological period which started with the confrontation between the Salpêtrière and Nancy schools and continued in the work of Freud, Janet and others.

But together with the concepts of hysteria and neurasthenia also survived a particular explanatory attitude, direct descendant of the physiopathological view. This attitude has sought to update itself according to experimental and ideological fashions and still lives on. Its persistence provides a partial explanation for the fact that the reflex model has survived transplantation onto scientific contexts (e.g. Pavlovianism) markedly different from the one it originated during the nineteenth century. Other movements, such as 'holistic' biologism have also left their mark on the physiopathological view of the neuroses: e.g. the neurovegetative dystonia of Eppinger's and Hess's is just a reformulation of the old nineteenth century model in terms of the totalistic concept of the body; the only difference being that the concept of neurovegetative dystonia was based on better knowledge of the autonomic nervous system and hence led to a generalization of the concept which had been considered as localized by nineteenth-century writers.

The so-called 'vasomotor and trophic neuroses'

The so-called 'vasomotor and trophic neuroses' were described and brought together by German physicians at the turn of the nineteenth century on account of their having a physiopathological common denominator. The identification of this factor was made possible by the growing knowledge on the vasomotor and trophic function of the autonomic nervous system; to this the work of Langley (1852–1925) greatly contributed.

The three nosological entities included by German authors in this group had been described for the first time not too long before: acrocyanosis (Raynaud, 1862), erythromelalgia (Weir-Mitchell, 1872) and angioneurotic oedema (Quincke, 1882).[307] To this core group of conditions, all characterized by vasomotor disturbances, dystrophic states were added such as scleroderma and atrophic and hypertrophic muscle disorders. Occasionally included also were diseases whose pathogenesis at the time merited a vasomotor explanation. For example, the vasomotor account of migraine offered by Du Bois-Reymond, Mollendorf and others and of angina pectoris suggested by Cahen, Traube and Landois, made possible their temporary inclusion into the group. The belief that Basedow's disease resulted from a vasomotor disorder also conferred upon this condition transient membership, which was lost when the new endocrine hypothesis was preferred. These oscillations can be illustrated by comparing two of Eulenburg's books: in the one published in 1875, he classified Basedow's disease, migraine, angina pectoris and germane conditions as 'vasomotor and trophic neurosis'[308]; in the monographic study of 1906[309] he excluded Basedow's disease, on the grounds that it was an endocrine condition and reduced the membership of the group to acrocyanosis, erythromelalgia, angioneurotic oedema and scleroderma.[310]

This group grew smaller as its components were gradually reclassified, and disappeared altogether the moment its remaining members ceased to be considered as neuroses. When the 'vasomotor and trophic neuroses' were first grouped, the term *neurosis* still used to mean 'functional nervous disease'. Under the impact of the psychological theories this meaning drastically changed during the early part of this century. In fact by the time Dubois coined the term *psychoneurosis* (in order to avoid confusion) the term neurosis had already acquired its present meaning.[311] In spite of this, writers at the beginning of the century continued referring to the 'trophic and vasomotor *neuroses*'. This particular usage, still present in our own day, is but a relic of a conceptual view which is no longer acceptable.

Endnotes

1 Bumke (1925), p. 1815
2 Temkin (1957)
3 The starting point of my study must be found in Laín Entralgo's view that the concept of neurosis reflects the successive medical views entertained during the nineteenth century (see Laín Entralgo, 1961, pp. 303–9; 368–71; 386–8)
4 See section on 'Cullen's concept of neurosis'
5 Eisenmann (1835), p. 60; Starck (1838), p. 1369; Ringseis (1841), p. 412
6 Platter's treatise (1602–3), where his account of traditional galenic medicine is contained, has three sections: I 'De functionum laesionibus'; II 'De doloribus'; III 'De vitiis'
7 Cullen (1786b), Vol. I, p. 249
8 Tissot (1782), Vol. I, Part I, p. X
9 Whytt (1767), p. 481. The sentence is taken from an appendix to the French rendition of Whytt's work on 'nervous diseases' which will be touched upon later on
10 On Willis see Feindel (1962), Isler (1965), Meyer & Hierons (1965) and López Piñero (1972)
11 The Amsterdam edition of the complete works by Willis (1682) has been consulted. *Cerebri anatome, nervorumque descriptio et usus* is printed in second place and keeps its own pagination (pp. 1–123). The 'animal spirits' are dealt with on pp. 30–1, 37, 48, 67
12 *Pathologiae cerebri et nervosi generis specimen in quo agitur de Morbis Convulsivis, et Scorbuto.* This is included in the Amsterdam edition of Willis's complete works third from the beginning, with its own pagination (pp. 1–146). The quotation on hysteria is on p. 70; Willis continued: 'Like other convulsive states, the affection vulgarly considered as hysterical is exclusively produced by explosions in the animal spirits. The forms of this disease can be told from each other and from other diseases in terms of the origin and extension of their morbid cause. Their more common origin is the head but they can also originate from uterine or other visceral alterations. As far as the extent of its spread is concerned the disease affects the internal nerves, namely those related to the viscera and the precordial parts, and also their prolongations thereby affecting the animal spirits contained therein, rarely it affects the spirits controlling the external nerves, cerebrum and cerebellum'
13 'The main symptoms of this disease (hypochondria) are spasmodic and depend directly upon disorders of the animal spirits and the nervous fluid

and not upon the visceral juices that serve to the digestion' (Willis, 1682, *Pathologiae cerebri*, p. 82). However Willis went on to say 'disorders of animal spirits and nervous fluid' may stem from 'spleen obstructions which impede its adequate function' (Willis, 1682, *Pathologiae cerebri*, p. 82)

14 *Affectionum quae dicuntur hystericae et hypochondriacae pathologia spasmodica vindicata. Contra Responsionem Epistolarem Nathanaelis Highmori, M.D. Cui accesserunt Exercitationes Medico-Physicae De sanguinis accensione, et motu musculari.* This is included in the Amsterdam Edition of Willis's complete works, fourth from the beginning, with its own pagination (pp. 1–41). The first section (pp. 1–17) is dedicated to the 'affections called hysterical or hypochondriacal'

15 *De anima brutorum quae hominis vitalis ac sensitiva est, exercitationes duae.* This is included in the Amsterdam edition of Willis's complete works fifth from the beginning, with its own pagination (pp. 1–210)

16 On Sydenham see Kleij (1930); Veith (1956); Schneck (1957); Laín Entralgo & Albarracín Teulón (1961); Dewhurst (1966); Albarracín (1973) and Bates (1977)

17 Sydenham (1682)

18 Sydenham (1848–50), Vol. II, p. 85

19 Sydenham (1848–50), Vol. II, p. 95

20 See Flashar (1966) and Fischer–Homberger (1970a, b)

21 Piso (1618)

22 I am referring to the attempt to substitute one for the many 'powers' of galenic physiology; in this Harvey and Descartes were interested (see Laín Entralgo, 1963, p. 33)

23 On Boerhaave, see Lindeboom (1968)

24 Boerhaave (1741), pp. 240–1

25 'Although such diseases are usually called hypochondriacal, when suffered by women are called hysterical for, once upon a time, they were considered as related to the uterus and were observed to worsen during menstruation and pregnancy. This notwithstanding it can be said that this condition originates exclusively from the increased irritability of the nerves and from the disordered movement of the animal spirits; because of this physicians have called it hypochondriacal disease sine materia... Sydenham offered the best description' (Van Swieten, 1755–73, Vol. III, p. 92). 'Hypochondria cum materia' Van Swieten touches upon in the same volume (pp. 481–8), following the views of Boerhaave

26 Oosterdijk Schacht (1767), Gorter (1750)

27 Lorry (1753–1757)

28 On Hoffmann, see King (1964), Rather (1973)

29 *Dissertatio medica sistens compendiosam et clinicam spasmodico-convulsivorum morborum praxin cum cautelis, primum edita anno 1707.* This is included in Hoffmann's complete works (1753), Vol. II, pp. 201–6. Other 'dissertationes practicae' by Hoffmann on the same topic are entitled *Dis. medica de vera morbi hypochondriaci sede, indole ac duratione* (Hoffmann's complete works (1753), pp. 207–15) and *Dis. medica, sistens affectum spasmodico-hypochondriacum inveteratum* (Hoffmann's complete works (1753), pp. 216–23)

30 On Stahl, see Turban (1950); Harms (1960); Gottlieb (1961); King (1964) and Rather (1973)

31 Stahl (1708), 'De passione hysterica', pp. 1110–17
32 Purcell (1702); Mandeville (1711). See Leigh (1961), pp. 19–28; Hunter & Macalpine (1963), pp. 288–91, 296
33 Du Moulin (1703)
34 Ridley (1738)
35 Pomme (1765), pp. 1–2
36 Blackmore (1725), Robinson (1729), Cheyne (1733), Flemyng (1740). On their work, see Leigh (1961), pp. 22–3, 28–31; Hunter & Macalpine (1963), pp. 319–24, 342–7, 351–4, 364–5; Skultans (1979), pp. 26–51; and also monographs on George Cheyne by Riddell (1922), Siddall (1942) and King (1974)
37 Perry (1755)
38 Whytt (1765)
39 Whytt (1767), pp. 479–577
40 Whytt (1767)
41 Blackmore (1725), p. V
42 Cheyne (1733), p. I
43 See French (1969)
44 Whytt (1765), p. III
45 Whytt (1765), p. 93
46 Adair (1786), p. 14
47 Whytt (1765). p. 102
48 Abercrombie (1829), Ollivier (1837), Romberg (1840–46). See Riese (1945), Haymaker (1953), Kolle (1956–63), McHenry (1969)
49 Tissot (1784). See Bucher (1958)
50 Boerhaave (1761). See Schulte (1959)
51 On Cullen and his work see Thomson, Thomson & Craigie (1832), Richardson (1890), Stapples (1897), Carlson & McFaden (1960), Risse (1974)
52 Cullen (1789), Vol. I, pp. LIX–LX (rejection of Boerhaave's humoralism); Vol. I, pp. LXVIII–LXX (views on Hoffmann's system); Vol. I, p. LXI (disdainful dismissal of Stahl's system)
53 See Rath (1954); Rath (1957)
54 On *more botanico*, see Most (1841), Diepgen (1941), Karst (1941), López Piñero (1961), Fischer-Homberger (1970a). Also see works on Sauvages and Linné by Berg (1956), Goerke (1966) and King (1966)
55 Cullen (1784), Vol. III, pp. 121–2
56 Cullen (1775), p. 193
57 Cullen (1784), Vol. III, p. 122
58 This corresponds to what Sauvages calls 'anepithymiae' and defines as 'marked weakness or unexplained suppression of sensitive appetites (without reduced awareness)'. The genera in this order are 'anorexia', 'adipsia' and 'anaphrodisia', and do not correspond to Cullen's 'comata'. They correspond well to Cl. VI, O. V
59 Cullen (1786b), Vol. I, p. 248
60 Cullen (1784), Vol. III, p. 122
61 Duncan (1778), Hosack (1821)
62 Crichton (1798)
63 Young (1813), Swediaur (1802)
64 Sagar (1771)

80 *Endnotes*

65 MacBride, D. (1813), Vol. I, p. 155
66 MacBride, D. (1813), Vol. I, p. 156
67 MacBride, D. (1813), Vol. I, p. 157
68 MacBride, D. (1813), Vol. I, p. 203
69 MacBride, D. (1813), Vol. I, p. 203–4
70 MacBride, D. (1813), Vol. I, p. 214–15
71 Blindness, impaired vision, deafness, impaired audition, anosmia, etc.
72 Anorexia, cynorexia, pica, polydipsia, satyriasis, etc.
73 MacBride, D. (1813), Vol. I, p. 222–3
74 Good (1817)
75 Darwin (1794–96), Sleigh (1825)
76 On Brownism see Hirschel (1846), Risse (1970) and Risse (1976)
77 Brown (1800), Vol. I, p. 39
78 On the relationship between British and German medicine during this period see Neuburger (1943) and Neuburger (1945)
79 For example in Fritsch's Leipzig printing of the German translations of the *First Lines* and of *Synopsis* the neologism 'neurosis' is replaced by 'Nervenkrankheit'. In Bosquillon's French rendition of the *First Lines* (1785–87) the terms 'névrose' and 'maladie nerveuse' are utilized exchangeably and so it is with the castilian translation by Piñera Siles (1789) that employs the term 'neurose o enfermedad nerviosa'
80 It has already been stated that the term 'nervous disease' had begun to develop its current meaning in the work of Abercrombie (1829), Ollivier (1837), Romberg (1840–46) and other founders of clinical neurology. It will soon be shown how in Georget's influential 1840 entry (written before 1828) 'neurosis' and 'nervous disease' are considered synonymous
81 See Neuburger (1943) and Rath (1954)
82 Fischer (1785)
83 Arnemann (1793)
84 Concerning Selle, see Karst (1941), pp. 26–9, and Heischkel (1956)
85 Selle (1773), p. 36
86 Selle (1773), p. 36
87 Selle (1781), Vol. II, p. 1
88 Selle (1781), Vol. II, p. 1
89 Selle (1773), p. 368
90 Selle (1773), p. 368
91 Selle (1773), p. 371
92 Selle (1781), Vol. II, p. 1 ss
93 Sagar (1771)
94 Of the many studies on Johann Peter Frank, only his autobiography with introduction and notes by Lesky (1969) will be mentioned here.
95 Frank (1792–1821)
96 Frank (1792–1821), Vol. I, p. XXVII
97 Frank (1851), p. 590
98 Frank (1851), p. 590
99 Daniel (1781–82)
100 Bang (1791)
101 Frank (1851), p. 592
102 Ploucquet (1793–97)
103 Ploucquet (1793–97), Vol. I, pp. 45–6

104 Ploucquet (1793–97), Vol. I, pp. 72 ss
105 Ploucquet (1793–97), Vol. I, p. 44
106 Ploucquet (1793–97)
107 Ploucquet (1793–97)
108 Thaer mentions this explicitly: Ploucquet (1793–97), Vol. I, p. 41
109 Cullen (1785)
110 Cullen (1785–87)
111 See Fischer (1925), Hirschfeld (1930), Diepgen (1938a), Galdston (1956), Liebbrand (1956), Risse (1972) and Risse (1976)
112 Ringseis (1841)
113 Ringseis (1841), pp. 409–33
114 On Reil, see Neuburger (1913), Boldt (1936), Petzold (1957) and Eulner (1960)
115 Reil (1800–15)
116 The main consequences of Kant's influence on Reil's vitalism can be listed thus:
   Matter is defined as 'what is contained in the phenomena which are perceived by the senses as objects in space'.
   Representations 'constitute a specific class of phenomena which must be differentiated from matter'.
   Force is defined as a subjective concept 'by means of which the relationship is expressed which links cause with effect and the properties of matter with the phenomena produced by them...'
   The identification by means of an analysis of phenomena, of two elementary features of the corporeal: composition or mixture ('Mischung') and form ('Form').
   Postulation of a 'vital principle' compatible with these ideas: 'Lebenskraft' refers not to a basic and unitary force but to the content of physico-chemical forces whose interaction gives origin to all vital manifestations. 'Irritability' is an expression or manifestation of 'Lebenskraft'
   Postulation of a distinction between two ways of becoming ill: 'diseases of the form' and 'diseases of the composition' which can be found in pure state or, more often, combined or changing into each other.
117 Reil (1800–15), Vol. IV, pp. 36–7
118 Reil (1800–15), Vol. I, p. 29
119 Reil (1800–15), Vol. I, p. 31
120 Reil (1800–15), Vol. I, p. 232–3
121 Neuburger (1913), p. 61
122 Reil (1800–15), Vol. I, p. 19
123 Reil (1800–15), Vol. I, p. 57
124 Reil (1800–15), Vol. IV, p. 36
125 See section on 'Pinel as the starting point of the anatomoclinical view of the neuroses'
126 Reil (1800–15), Vol. IV, p. 42
127 Reil (1800–15), Vol. IV, p. 42
128 Concerning Hufeland, see Diepgen (1938b), Berg (1962), Berghoff (1962) and Pfeifer (1968)
129 Hufeland (1836), p. 7
130 Hufeland (1836), p. 207

131 Hufeland (1836), p. 207 ss
132 Hufeland (1836), p. 208
133 Hufeland (1836), p. 208
134 Hufeland (1836), p. 209
135 See Karst (1941), pp. 41–4
136 Sachs (1828–29), p. 4
137 Sachs (1828–29), p. 28 ss
138 Sachs (1828–29), pp. 47–9
139 Sachs (1828–29), p. 53
140 Sachs (1828–29), pp.67–75
141 Hildenbrand (1816–25). See 2nd edn, 1833
142 Hildenbrand (1816–25), Vol. II, p. 20. See 2nd edn, 1833
143 Raimann (1816–17), pp. 526–7
144 Grossi (1831–32), Vol. III, pp. 178 ss
145 Conradi (1811)
146 Choulant (1831)
147 Choulant (1831)
148 Concerning Schoenlein, see Most (1841), Ebstein (1811) and Ackerknecht
     (1964)
149 Schoenlein (1839) and Schoenlein (1842)
150 Schoenlein (1839), Vol. I, p. 39
151 See works quoted in Endnote 111
152 Schoenlein (1839), Vol. I, p. 1
153 Schoenlein (1839), Vol. I, p. 40
154 Schoenlein (1839), Vol. I, pp. 40–1
155 Schoenlein (1839), Vol. I, p. 41
156 Schoenlein (1839), Vol. I, p. 41
157 Schoenlein (1839), Vol. I, p. 41
158 Schoenlein (1839), Vol. I, p. 41
159 Schoenlein (1839), Vol. IV, pp. 1–2
160 Schoenlein (1839), Vol. IV, p. 2
161 Schoenlein (1839), Vol. IV, p. 2
162 Schoenlein (1839), Vol. IV, pp. 2–3
163 Schoenlein (1839), Vol. IV, p. 31 ss
164 Schoenlein (1839), Vol. IV, p. 63 ss
165 Starck (1838). See Gemassner (1939) and Karst (1941), pp. 45–9
166 Eisenmann (1835)
167 See Maier (1948), pp. 32–5
168 Sobernheim (1837), p. 339
169 Sobernheim (1837), p. 339
170 Sobernheim (1837), pp. 340–1
171 Canstatt (1843–54)
172 Canstatt (1843–54), Vol. I, pp. 320–1
173 Canstatt (1843–54), Vol. I, p. 331–5
174 Canstatt (1843–54), *Suplement-Band*, p. 87
175 Hasse (1855)
176 Hasse (1855), p. 41
177 Concerning anatomoclinical medicine, see Laín Entralgo (1961), pp.
     179–364; Ackerknecht (1967c) and López Piñero (1973d)

178 Concerning Pinel, see Semelaigne (1912), Kavka (1949), Riese (1951), Lechler (1959), Veith (1960), Grange (1961), Woods & Carlson (1961), Marset (1970, 1971*a, b,* 1972, 1978)
179 Pinel (1818).
180 Pinel (1818), Vol I, p. XVI
181 Pinel (1818), Vol. III, p. 1 ss
182 Pinel (1818), Vol. III, p. 1
183 Pinel (1818), Vol. III, pp. 6–7
184 Pinel (1818), Vol. III, p. 7
185 Pinel (1818), Vol. III, pp. 8–9
186 Pinel (1818), Vol. III, pp. 4–5
187 Pinel (1818), Vol. III, pp. 294–5
188 On the doctrine of the 'passions' as an aetiological factor see Riese (1965) and Mullener (1966)
189 Richerand (1805–06)
190 Richerand (1822)
191 Richerand (1822), Vol. I, p. 1
192 Richerand (1822), Vol. I, pp. LX–LXI
193 Richerand (1822), Vol. I, p. LXVII
194 Richerand (1822), Vol. I, pp. LXVII–LXVIII
195 Richerand (1822), Vol. I, p. LXXIII
196 Duret (1815), Alibert (1817–25), Tourdes (1802)
197 Laennec (1819), Vol. I, p. 134
198 Georget (1840). On his scientific standing see Semelaigne (1930–32), Vol. I, pp. 188–96
199 Georget (1840), p. 29
200 Georget (1840), p. 29
201 See later the heading 'Broussais's *médecine physiologique*'
202 Georget (1840), p. 30
203 Georget (1840), p. 31
204 Georget (1840), p. 31. Georget considered 'nervous disease' and 'neurosis' as synonymous
205 Georget (1840), p. 31
206 Georget (1840), p. 31
207 On Foville, see Semelaigne (1930–32), Vol. I, pp. 250–6
208 Foville (1834)
209 Foville (1834), p. 55
210 Foville (1834), pp. 56–7
211 Foville (1834), p. 61
212 Foville (1834), p. 57
213 See below in sub-section 'Reflex functional nervous diseases'
214 Tardieu (1844), Monneret & Fleury (1836–46)
215 Tardieu (1844), p. 17
216 Monneret & Fleury (1836–46), Vol. VI, p. 209
217 Rosenthal (1878), Jaccoud (1872).
218 See below in sub-section 'The concept of spinal irritation'
219 Rosenthal (1878), p. 471
220 Rosenthal (1878), pp. 496–7
221 Rosenthal (1878), pp. 502–6

222 Jaccoud (1872), Vol. I, pp. 383–4
223 Louyer–Villermay (1816), Dubois (1837). On theories on hysteria during
    the first half of the nineteenth century see Bruttin's monograph (1969) and
    general works on hysteria by Cesbron (1909), Kraemer (1932),
    Delmas-Marsalet (1936), Kaech (1950), Wettley (1959) and Veith (1965)
224 Georget (1821), Voisin (1826)
225 Briquet (1859)
226 Briquet (1859), p. 661
227 Laín Entralgo (1961), pp. 365–436. See also López Piñero (1974)
228 This fact had already been remarked upon by Dubois (1849)
229 See López Piñero (1973b) and López Piñero (1974)
230 On Broussais, see Ackerknecht (1953)
231 Broussais (1821), Vol. I, pp. XXII, XXVII
232 See Beaugrand (1877)
233 Roche & Sanson (1836), Vol. I, p. 26
234 Roche & Sanson (1836), Vol. I, pp. 26–7
235 Roche & Sanson (1836), Vol. II, pp. 179–80
236 Roche & Sanson (1836), Vol. II, p. 180
237 Roche & Sanson (1836), Vol. II, p. 354
238 See López Piñero (1973b) and López Piñero (1974)
239 The term 'neurosis' vanished from Anglo-Saxon medical literature and was
    no longer mentioned in dictionaries or bibliographic sources such as
    Copland's *Medical Dictionary* (1844) or the first series of the *Index-Catalogue
    of the Library of the Surgeon-General's Office*, 1880–95. The term reappeared
    in the period during which the 'psychologization' of the concept took place;
    specially in the work of Daniel Hack Tuke. See López Piñero & Morales
    Meseguer (1968b)
240 Travers (1824)
241 Travers (1834)
242 The influence of Broussais on Travers had already been noticed by Baas
    (1876), p. 714. It is also patent in the chapter on 'irritation' of the *Lectures
    on the Principles and Practice of Surgery* by Astley Cooper (1837), where the
    great surgeon adopts the ideas of his own disciple
243 Cooper (1837)
244 Brodie (1837)
245 Williams (1843), Crawford & Tweedie (1845)
246 Abercrombie (1829), Bell (1830)
247 Player (1821)
248 Brown (1828)
249 Darwal (1829)
250 Ollivier (1837)
251 Teale (1829)
252 Tate (1830)
253 Parrish (1832)
254 Baas (1876), pp. 714–15
255 Turnbull (1837)
256 Griffin & Griffin (1834)
257 Stilling (1840), Türck (1843), Canstatt (1843–54)
258 Enz (1841)
259 Roux (1874)

260 Mayer (1860)
261 Leyden (1874–75)
262 Citation by Lereboullet (1883), p. 258
263 Ollivier (1837)
264 Valleix (1841), Monneret & Fleury (1836–46)
265 Fonssagrives (1856)
266 Valleix (1841), Leclerc (1852)
267 Armaingaud (1872), p. 251
268 Axenfeld (1863), Hammond (1871), Erb (1875), Erichsen (1975), Rosenthal (1878)
269 On the history of the reflex concept see Neuburger (1897), Fearing (1930), Hoff & Kellaway (1952), Canguilhem (1953), Fulton (1956), Liddell (1960) and Canguilhem (1964)
270 See the above section on 'The consolidation of the concept of nervous disease'
271 Whytt (1765)
272 On John Marshall Hall, see Erez-Federbusch (1963)
273 Hall (1841), pp. 198–200
274 Hall (1841), pp. 322–50
275 Hall (1855)
276 Stanley (1833)
277 Graves (1848)
278 Graves (1862)
279 Henoch (1845)
280 Romberg (1840–46)
281 Romberg (1857)
282 Jaccoud (1864), Jaccoud (1872)
283 Gull (1861)
284 Remak (1860)
285 On Leyden as a clinician, see Renvers (1902)
286 Leyden (1865)
287 Leyden (1870)
288 Leyden (1874–75), Vol. II, p. 207
289 On Brown-Séquard, see Olmsted (1946), Ruth (1946) and Lafont (1947)
290 Brown-Séquard (1868), Brown-Séquard (1878)
291 Valleix (1841)
292 Krishaber (1873)
293 Leven (1881)
294 For example in the neurological work by Ross (1883), Vol. II, pp. 173–7, 647–69
295 Kraus (1831), p. 44
296 Most (1836–37), Vol. II, p. 261
297 On Beard, see Rosenberg (1962) and Macmillan (1976)
298 Beard (1880), p. 15
299 Beard (1880)
300 Mitchell (1881)
301 Axenfeld (1863). The book by Silas Weir Mitchell (1883) on the treatment of neurasthenia appeared in French in the same year
302 Ziemssen (1887)
303 See López Piñero & Morales Meseguer (1964)

304 Charcot (1888–89)
305 Bouveret (1980), Levillain (1891), Mathieu (1892)
306 Bouchut (1877)
307 Raynaud (1862), Mitchell (1872), Quincke (1882)
308 Eulenburg (1875)
309 Eulenburg (1906*a*)
310 This was the volume on Neurology of *Die deutsche Klinik am Eingange des zwanzigsten Jahrhunderts* (1906) edited by Ernst von Leyden and Felix Klemperer. Cassirer (1906) who wrote the chapter on vasomotor neuroses, presented a summary of his own work including his monograph (1901). Migraine also became independent from the vasomotor neuroses during this period and deserved a separate chapter by Edinger (1906).
311 See López Piñero & Morales Meseguer (1968*b*)

References

Primary sources

Abercrombie, J. (1829). *Pathological and Practical Researches on Diseases of the Brain and the Spinal Cord*. Edinburgh: Waugh & Innes.

Adair, J. M. (1786). *Medical Cautions, for the Considerations of Invalids, those especially who resort to Bath*. Bath: Dodsley & Dilly.

Alibert, J. L. B. (1817–25). *Nosologie naturelle, ou les Maladies du Corps humaine distribuées par Familles*. Paris: Baillière.

Armaingaud, A. (1872). Du point douloureux apophysaire dans les névralgies et de l'irritation spinale. *Bordeux Médical*, 1, 251, 258, 267, 274, 283, 291.

Arnemann, J. (1793). *Synopsis nosologiae*. Gottingae: Vandenhoek et Ruprecht.

Axenfeld, A. (1863). Névroses (maladies nerveuses, névropathies). In *Elémens de Pathologie médicale*, vol. IV, ed. A. P. Requin, pp. 126–92. Paris: Germer-Baillière.

Bang, F. L. (1791). *Medizinische Praxis, systematisch erklärt und mit ausgewählten Krankengeschichten aus dem Tagebuche des Friedrich-Hospitals erläutert*. Kopenhagen: Prost.

Beard, G. M. (1880). *A Practical Treatise on Nervous Exhaustion (Neurasthenia). Its Causes, Symptoms and Sequences*. New York: Wood.

Bell, C. (1830). *The Nervous System of the Human Body... Appendix containing Cases and Letters of Consultation on Nervous Diseases...* London: Longman et al.

Blackmore, R. (1725). *A Treatise of the Spleen and Vapours: or Hypochondriacal and Hysterical Affections*. London: Pemberton.

Boerhaave, H. (1741). *Aphorismi de cognoscendis et curandis morbis in usum doctrinae domesticae digesti*. Venetiis: Basilius (1st edn, Leiden, 1709).

Boerhaave, H. (1761). *Praelectiones academicae de morbis nervorum quas ex auditorum manuscriptis collectas edi curavit Jacobus van Eems*. Lugduni Batavorum: van der Eyck & de Pecker.

Bouchut, E. (1877). *Du nervosisme aigu et chronique et des Maladies nerveuses*. Paris: Baillière.

Bouveret, L. (1890). *La neurasthénie, épuisement nerveux*. Paris: Baillière.

Briquet, P. (1859). *Traité clinique et thérapeutique de l'Hystérie*. Paris: Baillière.

Brochin, R. H. (1877). Nerveuses (maladies). In *Dictionnaire Encyclopédique des Sciences Médicales*, 2nd series, vol. XII, ed. A. Dechambre, pp. 332–91. Paris: Asselin & Masson.

Brodie, B. C. (1837). *Lectures Illustrative of Certain Local Nervous Affections*. London: Longman *et al*.

Broussais, F. J. V. (1821). *Examen des doctrines médicales et des systèmes de nosologie*. 2 vols. Paris: Méquignon-Marvis.

Brown, J. (1800). *Elementos de Medicina*. 2 vols. Madrid: Imprenta Real (1st edn, Edinburgh, 1780).

Brown, T. (1828). Irritation of the spinal nerves. *Glasgow Medical Journal*, 1, 131–60.

Brown-Séquard, C. E. (1868). *Lectures on the Diagnosis and Treatment of Functional Nervous Affections*. Philadelphia: Lippincott.

Brown-Séquard, C. E. (1878). *Lecciones sobre los Nervios vasomotores, la Epilepsia y las Acciones reflejas normales y morbosas*. Madrid: Sáiz (1st edn, Boston, 1857).

Canstatt, C. (1843–54). *Handbuch der medizinischen Klinik*. 2nd edn, 4 vols and Suplement-Band. Erlangen: Enke.

Cassirer, R. (1901). *Die vasomotorisch-trophischen Neurosen*. Berlin: Karger.

Cassirer, R. (1906). Die vasomotorisch-trophischen Neurosen. In *Die deutsche Klinik am Eingange des zwanzigsten Jahrhunderts*, vol. VI, part I, ed. E. von Leyden & F. Klemperer, pp. 719–43. Berlin & Wien: Urban & Schwarzenberg.

Charcot, J. M. (1888–89). *Leçons du Mardi à la Salpêtrière...Notes de Cours de M. M. Blin, Charcot et Colin*. Paris: Delahaye & Lecrosnier.

Cheyne, G. (1733). *The English Malady: or, a Treatise of Nervous Diseases of all Kinds, as Spleen, Vapours, Lowness of Spirits, Hypochondriacal and Hysterical Distempers*. London: Strahan & Leake.

Choulant, J. L. (1831). *Lehrbuch der speciellen Pathologie und Therapie des Menschen*. Leipzig: Voss.

Conradi, J. W. H. (1811). *Specielle Pathologie und Therapie*. Marburg: Krieger.

Cooper, A. P. (1837). *Lectures on the Principles and Practice of Surgery*. 8th edn. London: Cornish.

Copland, J. (1844). *A Dictionary of Practical Medicine*. 3 vols. London: Longman *et al*.

Crawford, J. & Tweedie, A. (1845). Inflammation. In *Cyclopaedia of Practical Medicine*, vol. II, ed. J. Forbes, A. Tweedie *et al*., pp. 694–804. London: Longman *et al*.

Crichton, A. (1798). *An Inquiry into the Nature and Origin of the Mental Derangement*. 2 vols. London: Cadell & Davies.

Cullen, W. (1775). *Apparatus ad Nosologiam Methodicam, seu Synopsis Nosologiae Methodicae in Usum Studiosorum*. Amstelodami: De Tournes (1st edn, Edinburgh, 1769).

Cullen, W. (1784). *First Lines of the Practice of Physic*. 4th edn, 4 vols. Edinburgh: Creech (1st edn, Edinburgh, 1777).

Cullen, W. (1785). *Institutions de Médecine pratique, traduites sur la quatrième et dernière Édition de l'Ouvrage anglois...par M. Pinel*. 2 vols. Paris & Versailles: Duplain & André.

Cullen, W. (1785–87). *Elémens de Médecine pratique...traduits de l'Anglois sur la quatrième et dernière édition, avec de Notes...par M. Bosquillon*. 2 vols. Paris: Barrois & Méquignon.

Cullen, W. (1786a). *Anfangsgründe der praktischen Arneykunst*. 4 vols. Leipzig: Fritsch.

Cullen, W. (1786b). *Kurzer Inbegriff der medizinischen Nosologie: oder systematische Einteilung der Krankheiten*. 2 vols. Leipzig: Fritsch.

Cullen, W. (1789). *Elementos de Medicina practica*. 4 vols. Madrid: Cano.

Daniel, C. F. (1781–82). *Systema aegritudinum conditum per nosologiam pathologiam...et symptomatologiam superstructas aetiologiae*. Lipsiae: Boehm.

Darwall, J. (1829). Observations upon some forms of spinal and cerebral irritation. *Midland Medical and Surgical Reporter Worcester*, 1, 229–40.

Darwin, E. (1794–96). *Zoonomia, or the Laws of Organic Life*. 2 vols. London: Johnson.

Dreyssig, F. W. (1796–98). *Handbuch der Pathologie der sogenannten chronischen Krankheiten*. 2 vols. Leipzig: Schwickert.

Dubois, E. F. (1837). *Histoire philosophique de l'Hypochondrie et de l'Hystérie*. Paris: Deville Cavellin.

Du Moulin, J. (1703). *Nouveau Traité du Rhumatisme, et des Vapeurs*. Paris: d'Houry.

Duncan, A. (1778). *De speciebus morborum constituendis*. Edinburgi.

Duret, F. J. J. (1815). *Tableau d'une Classification générale des Maladies*. Paris: Crochard.

Edinger, L. (1906). Von den Kopfschmerzen und der Migräne. In *Die deutsche Klinik am Eingange des zwanzigsten Jahrhunderts*, VI, 1, ed. E. von Leyden & J. Klemperer, pp. 31–50. Berlin & Wien: Urban & Schwarzenberg.

Eisenmann, G. (1835). *Die vegetativen Krankheiten und die entgiftende Heilmethode*. Erlangen: Palm & Enke.

Enz (1841). Bemerkungen in Betreff der Spinalirritation. *Medizinisches Correspondenblatt der württembergischer aerztlichen Vereinung*, Stuttgart, 11, 109.

Erb, W. (1875). Krankheiten des Rückenmarks und seiner Hüllen. In *Handbuch der speciellen Pathologie und Therapie*, XI, 2, ed. H. Ziemssen, pp. 1–404. Leipzig: Vogel.

Erichsen, J. E. (1875). *On Concussion of the Spine, Nervous Schock and other obscure Injuries of the Nervous System...* New York: Wood.

Eulenburg, A. (1875). Vasomotorisch-trophische Neurosen. In *Handbuch der speciellen Pathologie und Therapie*, XII, 2, ed. H. Ziemssen, pp. 1–175. Leipzig: Vogel.

Eulenburg, A. (1906a). Die Basedow'sche Krankheit nach ihrer heutigen Stande in Theorie und Praxis. In *Die deutsche Klinik am Eingange des zwanzigsten Jahrhunderts*, vol. VI, part I, ed. E. von Leyden & F. Klemperer, pp. 744–63. Berlin & Wien: Urban & Schwarzenberg.

Eulenburg, A. (1906*b*). Sexuale Neurasthenie. In *Die deutsche Klinik am Eingange des zwanzigsten Jahrhunderts*, vol. VI, part I, ed. E. von Leyden & F. Klemperer, pp. 162–206. Berlin & Wien: Urban & Schwarzenberg.

Fischer, I. (1785). *Genera morborum Culleni*. Gottingae.

Flemyng, M. (1740). *Neuropathia, seu de morbis hypochondriacis et hystericis libri III*. Eboraci: Ward & Chandler.

Fonssagrives, J. B. (1856). *Mémoire sur la Névralgie générale, et notamment sur celle d'Origine paludéenne*. Paris: Rignoux.

Foville, A. L. (1834). Névrose. In *Dictionnaire de Médecine et de Chirurgie Pratiques*, vol. XII, pp. 55–7. Paris: Gabon.

Frank, J. P. (1792–1821). *De curandis hominum morbis epitome*. 7 vols. Mannhemii: Schwan & Goetz; Tubingae: Cotta; Viennae: Schaumburg & Doll.

Frank, J. P. (1851). *Tratado de Medicina práctica*. Madrid: Compagni.

Fuchs, D. H. (1845). *Lehrbuch der speziellen Nosologie und Therapie*. Göttingen: Dieterich.

Georget, E. J. (1821). *De la physiologie du Système nerveux et spécialment du Cerveaux. Recherches sur les Maladies nerveuses en général, et en particulier sur le Siége, la Nature et le Traitement de l'Hystérie, de l'Hypochondrie, de l'Epilepsie et de l'Asthme convulsif*. 2 vols. Paris: Baillière.

Georget, E. J. (1840). Névroses. In *Dictionnaire de Médecine*, vol. XXV, pp. 27–41. Paris: Béchet.

Good, J. Mason (1817). *A Physiological System of Nosology*. London: Cox.

Gorter, J. de (1750). *Praxis medicae systema*. 2 vols. Harderovici: Wigmans.

Graves, R. J. (1848). *Clinical Lectures on the Practice of Medicine*. 2nd edn. Dublin: Fannin.

Graves, R. J. (1862). *Leçons de Clinique médicale...Ouvrage traduit et annoté par Jaccoud*. 2 vols. Paris: Delahaye.

Griffin, W. & Griffin, D. (1834). *Observations on the Functional Affections of the Spinal Cord and Ganglionic System of Nerves, in which their Identity with Sympathetic, Nervous, and Imitative Diseases is illustrated*. London: Burgess & Hill.

Grossi, E. (1831–32). *Opera medica posthuma*. Stuttgardtiae, Tubingae et Monachii.

Gull, W. W. (1861). On paralysis of the lower extremities consequent upon diseases of the bladder and kidneys. *Guy's Hospital Reports*, 3 series, 7, 313–31.

Hall, J. Marshall (1836). *Lectures on the Nervous System and its Diseases*. London: Sherwood, Gilbert & Piper.

Hall, J. Marshall (1841). *On the Diseases and Derangements of the Nervous System...* London: Baillière.

References 91

Hall, J. Marshall (1855). *Aperçu du Système spinal, ou de la Série des Actions réflexes dans leurs Applications à la Physiologie, à la Pathologie et Spécialement à l' Épilepsie.* Paris: Masson.

Hammond, W. A. (1871). *A Treatise on Diseases of the Nervous System.* New York: Appleton.

Hasse, K. E. (1855). Krankheiten des Nervenapparates. In *Handbuch der speciellen Pathologie,* vol. IV, ed. R. Virchow, pp. 1–686. Erlangen & Stuttgart: Enke.

Henoch, E. H. (1845). *Vergleichende Pathologie der Bewegungskrankheiten der Menschen und der Hausthiere.* Berlin: Hänel.

Highmore, N. (1660). *Exercitatione duae, prior de passione hysterica, altera de affectione hypochondriaca.* Oxoni: Lichfield.

Highmore, N. (1670). *De hysterica et hypochondriaca passione. Responsio epistolaris ad Doctorem Willis.* Londini: Clavel.

Hildenbrand, J. V. (1833). *Institutiones practico-medicae...* 2nd edn, 2 vols. Viennae: Heubner.

Hoffmann, F. (1753). *Operum omnium physico-medicorum supplementum secundum.* Genevae: De Tournes.

Hosack, D. (1821). *A System of Practical Nosology.* New York: Van Winkle.

Hufeland, C. W. (1836). *Enchiridion medicum oder Anleitung zum medizinischen Praxis.* Berlin: Jonas.

Jaccoud, D. (1864). *Etudes de Pathogénie et de Sémiotique. Les Paraplégies et l'Ataxie du Mouvement.* Paris: Delahaye.

Jaccoud, S. (1872). *Traité de Pathologie Interne.* 2nd edn, 2 vols. Paris: Delahaye.

Jahn, F. (1835). *System de Physiatrik.* Eisenach: Baerecke.

Kieser, D. G. (1817). *System der Medizin.* Halle: Schwetschke.

Kraus, L. A. (1831). *Kritisch-etymologisches medicinisches Lexikon...* Theil 1. Wien: Haykul & Lechner.

Krishaber, M. (1873). Cérébro-cardiaque (Névropathie). In *Dictionnaire Encyclopédique des Sciences Médicales,* series 1, vol. XIV, ed. A. Dechambre, pp. 100–42. Paris: Masson & Asselin.

Laennec, R. T. H. (1819). *De l'Auscultation médiate, ou Traité du diagnostic des Maladies du poumon et du coeur fondé principalment sur un nouveau Moyen d'exploration.* 2 vols. Paris: Brosson & Chaudé. (2nd edn, Paris, 1826).

Leclerc, M. M. J. (1852). *De la Névralgie générale.* Paris.

Lereboullet, L. (1883). Spinale (Irritation). In *Dictionnaire Encyclopédique des Sciences Médicales,* séries 3, vol. XI, ed. A. Dechambre, pp. 252–69. Paris: Masson & Asselin.

Leven, G. (1881). Gastralgie. In *Dictionnaire Encyclopédique des Sciences Médicales,* series 4, vol. VII, ed. A. Dechambre, pp. 2–13. Paris: Masson & Asselin.

Levillain, F. (1891). *La Neurasthénie, Maladie de Beard.* Paris: Maloine.

Leyden, E. v. (1860). Ueber Reflexlähmungen. In *Sammlung Klinische Vorträge. Innere Medizin*, vol. 1, ed. R. von Volkmann, pp. 1–22. Leipzig: Breitkopf & Härtel.

Leyden, E. v. (1865). *De paraplegiis urinariis commentatio*. Regimonti: Hartung.

Leyden, E. v. (1874–76). *Klinik der Rückenmarks-Krankheiten*. 2 vols. Berlin: Hirschwald.

Linné, C. (1763). *Genera morborum in auditorum usu*. Upsaliae: Steinert.

Lorry, A. C. (1753–1757). *De melancholia et de morbis melancholicis*. Lutetiae Parisiorum: Cavelier.

Louyer-Villermay, J. B. (1816). *Traité des Maladies nerveuses ou vapeurs, et particulièrement de l'Hystérie et de l'Hypocondrie*. 2 vols. Paris: Méquignon.

MacBride, D. (1813). *Introducción metódica a la Medicina teórica y práctica*. Madrid: Repullés (1st edn, London, 1772).

Mandeville, B. (1711). *A Treatise of the Hypochondriack and Hysterick Passions*...London: Learb.

Mathieu, A. (1892). *Neurasthénie (Epuisement nerveux)*. Paris: Reuff.

Mayer, A. (1860). Die Lehre der sogennanten Spinal-Irritation in der letzten zehn Jahre. *Archiv der Heilkunde*, 1, 121–56.

Mitchell, S. W. (1872). Clinical lecture on certain painful affections of the feet. *Philadelphia Medical Times*, 3, 81, 113.

Mitchell, S. Weir (1881). *Lectures on the Diseases of the Nervous System, especially in Women*. Philadelphia: Lea.

Mitchell, S. Weir (1883). *Du Traitement méthodique de la Neurasthénie et de quelques formes d'Hystérie*. Paris: Bethier.

Monneret, E. & Fleury, L. (1836–46). *Compendium de Médecine pratique*. 8 vols. Paris: Béchet.

Most, G. F. (1836–37). *Encyclopädie des gesammten medicinischen und chirurgischen Praxis*...2nd edn, 2 vols. Leipzig: Brockhaus.

Ollivier (d'Angers), C. P. (1837). *De la Moëlle épinière et de ses Maladies*. 3rd edn, 2 vols. Paris: Méquignon-Marvis.

Oosterdijk Schacht, J. (1767). *Institutiones medicinae practicae*. 2nd edn, Trajecti ad Rhenum: Paddenburg (1st edn, Utrecht, 1747).

Parrish, I. (1832). Remarks on spinal irritation as connected with nervous diseases. *American Journal of Medical Sciences*, 10, 293–314.

Perry, C. (1755). *A Mechanical Account and Explication of the Hysteric Passion*. London.

Pinel, P. (1818). *Nosographie philosophique, ou la Méthode de l'Analyse appliquée à la Médecine*. 6th edn, 3 vols. Paris: Brosson. (1st edn, Paris, 1798).

Piso, C. (1618). *Selectionum observationum et consiliorum de praeteritis hactenus morbis, effectibusque praeter naturam ab aqua, seu serosa colluvie et dilluvie, ortis, liber singularis*. Ponte ad Monticulum: Mercator.

Platter, F. (1602–3). *Praxeos seu de cognoscendis, praecavendis, curandisque affectibus homini incommodantibus tractatus.* 3 vols. Basileae: Waldkirch.

Player, R. F. (1821). On irritation of the spinal nerves. *Quarterly Journal of Science, Literature and the Arts,* 14, 296.

Ploucquet, W. G. (1793–97). *Delineatio systematis nosologici naturae accomodati.* 4 vols. Tübingae: Heerbrandt.

Pomme, P. (1765). *Traité des Affections vapoureuses des deux Sexes.* Lyon: Duplain.

Purcell, J. (1702). *A Treatise of Vapours, or Hysterick Fits.* London: Newman & Cox.

Quincke, H. I. (1882). Ueber akutes umschriebenes Hautödem. *Monatschrift für praktische Dermatologie,* 1, 129–31.

Raimann, J. N. (1816–17). *Handbuch der speziellen medizinischen Pathologie und Therapie.* Wien: Heubner & Volke.

Raynaud, M. (1862). *De l'Asphysie locale et de la Gangrène symétrique des extrémités.* Paris.

Reil, J. C. (1800–15). *Ueber die Erkenntnis und Kur der Fieber.* 5 vols. Wien: Ghelen.

Remak, R. (1860). Ueber die durch Neuritis bedingten Lähmungen, Neuralgien und Krämpfe. *Allgemeine medizinische Central-Zeitung,* 29, 12.

Richerand, A. (1805–6). *Nosographie et Thérapeutique chirurgicales.* 3 vols. Paris: Caille & Ravier.

Richerand, A. (1822). *Nosographia y Terapéutica quirúrgicas.* 4 vols. Madrid: Aribau. (Translation of the fourth French edn, Paris, 1815).

Ridley, H. (1738). *Observations quaedam medico-practicae et physiologicae.* Lugduni Batavorum: Langerak & Ruck.

Ringseis, J. N. (1841). *System der Medizin.* Regensburg: Manz.

Robinson, N. (1729). *A New System of the Spleen, Vapours, and Hypochondriack Melancholy. Wherein all the Decays of the Nerves, and Lownesses of the Spirits, are mechanically Accounted for.* London: Bettesworth, Innys & Rivington.

Roche, L. C. & Sanson, L. J. (1836). *Nuevos elementos de patología médico-quirúrgica.* 5 vols. Madrid: Fuentenebro. (1st edn, Paris, 1825–28).

Romberg, M. H. (1840–46). *Lehrbuch der Nervenkrankheiten des Menschen.* 2 vols. Berlin: Duncker.

Romberg, M. H. (1857). *Pathologie und Therapie der Sensibilität- und Mobilitätneurosen.* Berlin: Hirschwald.

Rosenthal, M. (1878). *Tratado clínico de las enfermedades del sistema nervioso.* Madrid: Teodoro. (1st edn, Erlangen, 1870).

Ross, J. (1883). *A Treatise of the Diseases of the Nervous System.* 2nd edn, 2 vols. London: Churchill.

Roux, P. C. C. (1874). *Étude historique et critique sur l'Irritation spinale.* Paris.

94   References

Sachs, L. W. (1828–29). *Handbuch des naturlichen System der praktischen Medizin*. Leipzig.

Sagar, J. B. M. (1771). *Systhema morborum symptomaticum, secundum classes, ordines et genera, cum characteribus propositum*. Viennae: Kraus.

Sauvages, F. B. (1763). *Nosologia methodica sistens morborum classes, genera et species juxta Sydenhami mentem et botanicorum ordinem*. 5 vols. Amstelodami: de Tournes.

Schoenlein, J. L. (1839). *Allgemeine und specielle Pathologie und Therapie nach dessen Vorlesungen niedergeschrieben und heraugegeben von einigen seiner Zuhörer*. 4 vols. St. Gallen–Leipzig.

Schoenlein, J. L. (1842). *Klinische Vorträge in dem Charité-Krankenhaus zu Berlin*. Berlin: Veit.

Seeligmueller, O. L. G. A. (1888). Neurastenia. In *Tratado Enciclopédico de Patología Médica y Terapéutica*, vol. VIII, ed. H. Ziemssen, pp. 907–31. Madrid: Rivadeneyra. (1st edn, Leipzig, 1883).

Selle, C. G. (1773). *Rudimenta pyretologiae methodicae*. Berolini: Himburg.

Selle, C. G. (1781). *Medicina clinica, oder Handbuch der medizinischen Praxis*. Berlin: Himburg.

Sleigh, W. W. (1825). *Science of Surgery*. London: Anderson.

Sobernheim, J. F. (1837). *Praktische Diagnostik der inneren Krankheiten*. Berlin: Schüppel.

Stahl, G. E. (1708). *Theoria medica vera*. Halae: Lit. Orphanotrophei.

Stanley, E. (1833). On the irritation of the spinal cord and its nerves in connexion with diseases of the kidneys. *Medical & Chirurgical Transactions*, **18**, 260.

Starck, K. W. (1838). *Allgemeine Pathologie, oder allgemeine Naturlehre der Krankheit*. Leipzig: Breitkopf & Härtel.

Stilling, B. (1840). *Physiologische, pathologische und medicinisch-praktische Untersuchungen über die Spinalirritation*. Leipzig: Wigand.

Swediaur, F. X. (1802). *Novum nosologiae methodicae systema*. Paris.

Sydenham, T. (1682). *Dissertatio epistolaris ad G. Cole de observationis nuperis circa curationem variolarum confluentium, necnon de affectione hysterica*. Londini: Kettilby.

Sydenham, T. (1848–50). *The Works...translated from the Latin Edition of Dr. Greenhill with a Life of the Author, by R. G. Latham*. 2 vols. London: Sydenham Society.

Tardieu, A. A. (1844). *Jusqu'à quel point le diagnostic anatomique peut-il éclarer le Traitement des Névroses?* Paris (Thèse d'agregation).

Tate, G. (1830). *A Treatise of Hysteria*. London: Highley.

Teale, T. P. (1829). *A Treatise of Neuralgic Disease dependent upon Irritation of the Spinal Marrow and Ganglia of Sympathetic Nerves*. London: Highley.

Tissot, S. A. (1784). *Traité des Nerfs et de leurs Maladies*. 2 Vols in 4 parts, Lausanne: s.i. (1st edn, Paris, 1778–80).

Todd, R. B. (1861). *Clinical Lectures*. 2nd edn, London: Churchill.

Tourdes, J. T. (1802). *Esquisse d'une Système de Nosologie, fondé sur la Physiologie et la Thérapeutique*. Strasbourg.

References 95

Tourtelle, E. (1799). Elémens de médecine théorique et pratique. 2 vols. Strasbourg: Eck.

Travers, B. (1824). An Inquiry concerning that Disturbed State of the Vital Functions usually denominated Constitutional Irritation. London: Longman et al.

Travers, B. (1834). A further Inquiry concerning Constitutional Irritation and the Pathology of the Nervous System. London: Longman et al.

Türck, L. (1843). Abhandlung über Spinalirritation nach eigenen, grösstentheils in wiener allgemeinen Krankenhause angestellten Beobachtungen. Wien: Braunmüller & Seidel.

Turnbull, A. (1837). A Treatise on Painful and Nervous Diseases. London: Churchill.

Valleix, F. L. I. (1841). Traité des névralgies ou Affections douloureuses des Nerfs. Paris: Baillière.

Van Swieten, G. (1755–1773). Commentaria in Hermanni Boerhaave Aphorismos de cognoscendis et curandis morbis. 5 vols. Parisiis: Cavelier (1st edn, Leiden, 1742–46).

Vogel, R. A. (1764). Definitiones genera morborum. Gottingae.

Voisin, F. (1826). Des Causes morales et physiques des Maladies mentales et de quelques autres Affections nerveuses, telles que l'Hystérie, la Nymphomanie et la Satyriasis. Paris: Baillière.

Walton, G. L. (1883). Spinal irritation; probable cerebral origin of the symptoms sometimes classed under this head. Boston Medical and Surgical Journal, 109, 601–3.

Whytt, R. (1765). Observations on the Nature, Causes and Cure of those Disorders which are commonly called Nervous, Hypochondriac, or Hysteric. Edinburgh: Becket & Du Hondt.

Whytt, R. (1767). Les Vapeurs et Maladies nerveuses, hypochondriaques ou hystériques. Paris: Vincent.

Williams, C. J. B. (1843). Principles of Medicine: comprising General Pathology and Therapeutics... London: Churchill.

Willis, T. (1682). Opera omnia. Amstelodami: Wetstenius.

Young, T. (1813). An Introduction to Medical Literature, including a System of Practical Nosology. London: Underwood.

Ziemssen (1887). Die Neurasthenie und ihre Behandlung. Leipzig: Vogel.

Selected references

Abricosoff, G. (1897). L'Hystérie aux XVIIe et XVIIIe Siècles (Etude historique et bibliographique). Paris: Steinheil.

Ackerknecht, E. H. (1953). Broussais, or a forgotten medical revolution. Bulletin of the History of Medicine, 27, 320–43.

Ackerknecht, E. H. (1964). Johann Lucas Schoenlein (1793–1864). Journal of the History of Medicine, 19, 131–8.

Ackerknecht, E. H. (1967a). Kurze Geschichte der Medizin. 2nd edn. Stuttgart: Enke.

Ackerknecht, E. H. (1967*b*). *Kurze Geschichte der Psychiatrie.* 2nd edn. Stuttgart: Enke.

Ackerknecht, E. H. (1967*c*). *Medicine at the Paris Hospital, 1794–1848.* Baltimore: The Johns Hopkins Press.

Albarracín, A. (1973). Sydenham. In *Historia Universal de la Medicina,* vol. V, ed. P. Laín Entralgo, pp. 297–307. Barcelona: Salvat.

Aschaffenburg, G. (1915). Die Wandlungen des Neurastheniebegriffes. *Schmidt's Jahrbuch,* **323,** vol. comp., 43–52.

Baas, J. H. (1876). *Grundriss der Geschichte der Medizin und des heilenden Standes.* Stuttgart: Enke.

Baruk, H. (1967). *La Psychiatrie française de Pinel à nos Jours.* Paris: Presses Universitaires de France.

Bates, D. G. (1977). Sydenham and the medical meaning of method. *Bulletin of the History of Medicine,* **51,** 324–38.

Beaugrand, E. (1877). Louis-Charles Roche. In *Dictionnaire Encyclopédique des Sciences Médicales,* séries 3, vol. V, ed. A. Dechambre, pp. 95–7. Paris: Masson & Asselin.

Berg, A. (1962). Hufeland, Arzt zwischen den Zeiten. *Medizinische Monatsschrift,* **16,** 551–7.

Berg, F. (1956). Linné et Sauvages. Les rapports entre leurs systèmes nosologiques. *Lychnos,* 31–54.

Berghoff (1962). Christoph Wilhelm Hufeland, ein Pionier der prophylaktischen Medizin. *Prophylaxis und Therapie,* **1,** 2–4.

Boldt, A. (1936). *Ueber die Stellung und Bedeutung der 'Rapsodien über die Anwendung der psychische Curmethode auf Geisteszerrüttungen' von Johann Christian Reil (1759–1818) in der Geschichte der Psychiatrie.* Berlin: Ebering.

Boring, E. G. (1950). *A History of Experimental Psychology.* 2nd edn. New York: Appleton-Century-Crofts.

Brain, R. (1963). The concept of hysteria in the time of Harvey. *Proceedings of the Royal Society of Medicine,* **56,** 317–24.

Bruttin, J. M. (1969). *Différentes Théories sur l'Hystérie dans la première Moitié du XIX* *Siècle.* Zürich: Juris (Medizinhistorisches Institut der Universität Zürich).

Bucher, H. W. (1958). *Tissot und sein 'Traité des nerfs'. Ein Beitrag zur Medizingeschichte der schweizerischen Aufklärung.* Zürich: Juris (Medizinhistorisches Institut der Universität Zürich).

Bumke, O. (1925). Die Revision der Neurosen-frage. *München medizinische Wochenschrift,* **72,** 1815–18.

Canguilhem, G. (1953). *La Formation du Concept du Réflexe aux XVII* *et XVIII* *Siècles.* Paris: Presses Universitaires de France.

Canguilhem, G. (1964). Le concept du réflexe au XIX³ siècle. In *Von Boerhaave bis Berger,* ed. K. E. Rothschuch, pp. 157–67. Stuttgart: Fischer.

Carlson, E. T. & McFaden, R. B. (1960). Dr William Cullen on mania. *American Journal of Psychiatry*, 117, 463–5.

Cesbron, H. (1909). *Histoire critique de l'Hystérie*. Paris: Asselin & Houzeau.

Chabbert, P. (1966). Philippe Pinel à Paris (jusqu'à sa nomination à Bicêtre). In *Aktuelle Probleme aus der Geschichte der Medizin*, pp. 589–95. Basel & New York: Karger.

Delmas-Marsalet, P. (1936). L'évolution des idées sur l'hystérie. *Journal Médical de Bordeaux*, 113, 195–202.

De Saussure, R. (1950). French psychiatry in the eighteenth century. *Ciba Symposium*, 11, 1222–52.

Dewhurst, K. (1966). *Dr Thomas Sydenham (1624–1689). His Life and Original Writings*. Berkeley & Los Angeles: University of California Press.

Dezeimeris, J. E., Ollivier, C. P. & Raige-Delorme, J. (1829–1839). *Dictionnaire historique de la Médicine ancienne et moderne*. 4 vols. Paris: Béchet.

Diepgen, P. (1938a). Alte und neue Romantik in der Medizin. In *Medizin und Kultur*, pp. 224–42. Stuttgart: Enke.

Diepgen, P. (1938b). C. W. Hufeland und die Medizin seiner Zeit. In *Medizin und Kultur*, pp. 210–23. Stuttgart: Enke.

Diepgen, P. (1941). Die Stellung der nosologische Systeme in der Geschichte der Medizin. *Archiv für Geschichte der Medizin*, 34, 61–7.

Dubois, E. F. (1849). Éloge de F. J. V. Broussais. *Mémoires de l'Académie de Médecine, Paris*, 14, I–XXVIII.

Dukor, B. (1950). Die 'Hysterie' in moderner Auffassung. *Ciba Zeitschrift*, 10, 4427–34.

Ebstein, E. (1911). J. L. Schönlein. *Archiv für Geschichte der Medizin*, 4, 449–52.

Erez-Federbusch, R. (1963). *Marshall Hall, 1797–1857, Physiologe und Praktiker*. Zürich: Juris (Medizinhistorisches Institut der Universität Zürich).

Eulner, H. H. (1960). Johann Christian Reil (1759–1813). *Neue Zeitschrift für aerztliche Fortbildung*, 49, 472–4.

Fearing, F. (1930). *Reflex Action. A Study in the History of Physiological Psychology*. Baltimore: William & Wilkins.

Feindel, W. (1962). Thomas Willis (1621–1675), the founder of neurology. *Canadian Medical Association Journal*, 87, 289–96.

Fischer, W. (1926). *Die Krankheitsanschauungen der Romantik*. Rostock.

Fischer-Homberger, E. (1970a). Eighteenth century nosology and its survivors. *Medical History*, 14, 397–403.

Fischer-Homberger, E. (1970b). *Hypochondrie. Melancholie bis Neurose. Krankheiten und Zustandbilder*. Bern: Huber.

Fischer-Homberger, E. (1975). *Die traumatische Neurose. Vom somatischen zum sozialen Leiden*. Bern: Huber.

98   *References*

Flashar, H. (1966). *Melancholie und Melancholiker in den medizinischen Theorien der Antike.* Berlin: W. de Gruyter.

Foucault, M. (1961). *Histoire de la Folie à l'Age classique.* Paris: Plon.

French, R. K. (1969). *Robert Whytt, the Soul, and Medicine.* London: The Wellcome Institute of the History of Medicine.

Fulton, J. F. (1956). Reflections on the History of Reflex Action. *Archivo Iberoamericano de Historia de la Medicina,* **8**, 27–32.

Galdston, I. (1956). The romantic period in medicine. *Bulletin of the New York Academy of Medicine,* **32**, 346–52.

Gemassner, J. (1939). *Die Pathologie von Karl Wilhelm Stark.* Berlin-Charlottenburg: Hoffmann.

Goerke, H. (1966). *Carl von Linné, Arzt, Naturforscher, Systematiker, 1707–1778.* Stuttgart: Wissenschaftliche Verlagsgesellschaft.

Gottlieb, B. J. (1961). *G. E. Stahl: Ueber die mannifaltigen Einfluss der Gemüthsbewegungen auf den menschlichen Körper (Halle, 1695) und drei weitere Arbeiten.* Leipzig: Barth.

Grange, K. M. (1961). Pinel and eighteenth-century psychiatry. *Bulletin of the History of Medicine,* **35**, 442–53.

Harms, E. (1960). Georg Ernst Stahl. *American Journal of Psychiatry,* **117**, 366–7.

Haymaker, W., ed. (1953). *The Founders of Neurology. One Hundred and Thirty Three Biographical Sketches.* Springfield: Thomas.

Heischkel, E. (1956). Die Medizin der Goethezeit. *Ciba Zeitschrift (Wehr/Baden),* **7**, 2646–76.

Hirsch, A., ed. (1929–1935). *Biographisches Lexikon der hervorragenden Aerzte aller Zeiten und Völker.* 2nd edn, 5 vols. + vol. comp. Berlin & Wien: Urban & Schwarzenberg.

Hirschel, B. (1846). *Geschichte des brownschen Systems und der Erregungstheorie.* Dresden & Leipzig: Arnold.

Hirschfeld, E. (1930). Romantische Medizin. *Kyklos,* **3**, 1–89.

Hoff, E. & Kellaway, P. (1952). The early history of reflex. *Journal of the History of Medicine,* **7**, 211–49.

Hunter, R. & Macalpine, I. (1963). *Three Hundred Years of Psychiatry.* London: Oxford University Press.

Irsay, S. d' (1928). Der philosophische Hintergrund der Nervenphysiologie im 17. und 18. Jahrhundert. *Archiv für Geschichte der Medizin,* **20**, 181–97.

Isler, H. (1965). *Thomas Willis. Ein Wegbereiter der modernen Medizin, 1621–1675.* Stuttgart: Wissenschaftliche Verlagsgesellschaft (Medizinhistorisches Institut der Universität Zürich).

Kaech, R. (1950). Die somatische Auffassung der Hysterie. *Ciba Zeitschrift (Basel),* **10**, 4406–18.

Karst, W. (1941). *Zur Geschichte der natürlichen Krankheitssysteme.* Berlin: Ebering.

References 99

Kavka, J. (1949). Pinel's conception of the psychopathic state; an historical critique. *Bulletin of the History of Medicine*, 23, 461–8.

Kenyon, F. E. (1965). Hypochondriasis: a survey of some historical, clinical and social aspects. *British Journal of Medical Psychology*, 38, 117–33.

King, L. S. (1964). Stahl and Hoffmann: a study in eighteenth century animism. *Journal of the History of Medicine*, 19, 118–30.

King, L. S. (1966). Boissier de Sauvages and 18th Century Nosology. *Bulletin of the History of Medicine*, 40, 43–51.

King, L. S. (1974). George Cheyne, mirror of eighteenth century medicine. *Bulletin of the History of Medicine*, 48, 517–39.

Kleij, J. van der (1930). Thomas Sydenham (1624–1689) en zijn verhandeling over de hysterie. *Bijdragen tot de Geschiedenis der Geneeskunde*, 10, 271–8.

Kolle, K., ed. (1956–1963). *Grosse Nervenaerzte*. 3 vols. Stuttgart: Thieme.

Kraemer, R. (1932). *Der Wandel in den wissenschaftlichen Anschauungen über Hysterie unter besonderer Berücksichtigung der letzten Jahrzehnte*. Würzburg.

Laehr, H. (1900). *Die Literatur der Psychiatrie, Neurologie und Psychologie von 1459–1799*. 3 vols. Berlin: Reimer.

Lafont, J. (1947). Brown-Séquard (1817–1894). *Progrès Médical*, 75, 637–8.

Laignel-Lavastine, M. & Vinchon, J. (1931). *Les Maladies de l'Esprit et leurs Médecins du XVIᵉ au XIXᵉ Siècles. Les étapes des Connaissances psychiatriques de la Renaissance à Pinel*. Paris: Maloine.

Laín Entralgo, P. (1950). *Introducción histórica al estudio de la Patología psicosomática*. Madrid: Paz Montalvo.

Laín Entralgo, P. (1961). *La Historia clínica. Historia y teoría del relato patográfico*. 2nd edn. Barcelona: Salvat.

Laín Entralgo, P. (1963). *Historia de la Medicina moderna y contemporánea*. 2nd edn. Barcelona: Científico-Médica.

Laín Entralgo, P. & Albarracín Teulón, A. (1961). *Sydenham*. Madrid: C.S.I.C.

Lechler, W. (1959). *Philippe Pinel. Seine Familie, seine Jugend- und Studienjahre, 1745–1778*... München (doctoral dissertation).

Leibbrand, W. (1956). *Die spekulative Medizin der Romantik*. Hamburg: Claassen.

Leibbrand, W. & Wettley, A. (1961). *Der Wahnsinn. Geschichte der abendländischen Psychopathologie*. Freiburg & München: Alber.

Leigh, D. (1961). *The Historical Development of British Psychiatry*, vol. 1, 18th & 19th C. Oxford: Pergamon Press.

Lesky, E. (1965). *Die wiener medizinische Schule im 19. Jahrhundert*. Graz & Köln: Böhlau.

Lesky, E. (1969). *Johann Peter Frank: Seine Selbstbiographie*...*eingeleitet und mit Erläuterungen versehen*... Bern: Huber.

Liddell, E. G. T. (1960). *The Discovery of Reflexes*. Oxford: Clarendon Press.

Lindeboom, G. A. (1968). *Herman Boerhaave. The Man and his Work*. London: Methuen.

López Piñero, J. M. (1961). Los sistemas nosológicos del siglo XVIII. *Archivo Iberoamericano de Historia de la Medicina*, **13**, 65–93.

López Piñero, J. M. (1972). El primer sistema médico moderno: la iatroquímica de la segunda mitad del siglo XVII. *Medicina Española*, **67**, 164–73, 228–37.

López Piñero, J. M. (1973*a*). Clínica y patología de la Ilustración. Europa Latina. In *Historia Universal de la Medicina*, vol. **5**, ed. P. Laín Entralgo, pp. 73–84. Barcelona: Salvat.

López Piñero, J. M. (1973*b*). *John Hughlings Jackson (1835–1911). Evolucionismo y neurología*. Madrid: Moneda y Crédito.

López Piñero, J. M. (1973*c*). Las neurosis en la 'Psychiatrie' de Kraepelin. In *Actas de VI Congreso Español de Historia de la Medicina*, pp. 55–61. Granada: Sociedad Española de Historia de la Medicina.

López Piñero, J. M. (1973*d*). Patología y clínica en el Romanticismo. Europa Latina. In *Historia Universal de la Medicina*, vol. **5**, ed. P. Laín Entralgo, pp. 255–65. Barcelona: Salvat.

López Piñero, J. M. (1974). Patología y medicina interna (durante la segunda mitad del siglo XIX). In *Historia Universal de la Medicina*, vol. **6**, ed. P. Laín Entralgo, pp. 123–55, 171–2. Barcelona: Salvat.

López Piñero, J. M. & Morales Meseguer, J. M. (1963). La mentalidad fisiopatológica ante el concepto de neurosis. *Archivo Iberoamericano de Historia de la Medicina*, **15**, 121–56.

López Piñero, J. M. & Morales Meseguer, J. M. (1964). Neurosis y psicoterapia en la obra de Charcot. *Asclepio*, **16**, 29–95.

López Piñero, J. M. & Morales Meseguer, J. M. (1965–66). Los comienzos de la psicoterapia contemporánea: W. B. Carpenter, D. Hack Tuke y J. Hughes Bennet. *Medicina Española*, **54**, 320–33.

López Piñero, J. M. & Morales Meseguer, J. M. (1967). Hipnotismo y psicoterapia en la medicina alemana de finales del siglo XIX. In *Melémata, Festschrift für Werner Leibbrand zum seibzigsten Geburtstag*, pp. 75–94. Mannheim: Boehringer.

López Piñero, J. M. & Morales Meseguer, J. M. (1968*a*). El punto de partida de la obra de Pierre Janet acerca de la neurosis y la psicoterapia. *Asclepio*, **20**, 67–98.

López Piñero, J. M. & Morales Meseguer, J. M. (1968*b*). *Neurosis y psicoterapia. Un estudio histórico*. Madrid: Espasa Calpe.

López Piñero, J. M. & Morales Meseguer, J. M. (1968–69). La Escuela de Nancy en la historia de la psicoterapia y del concepto de neurosis. *Episteme*, **2**, 179–99, **3**, 137–59.

Macmillan, M. B. (1976). Beard's concept of neurasthenia and Freud's concept of the actual neuroses. *Journal of the History of Behavioral Sciences*, **12**, 376–90.

References 101

Maier, J. S. (1948). *Beitrag zur Geschichte der Neurosebegriffes.* Erlangen (doctoral dissertation).
Maier, J. S. (1948). Beitrag zur Geschichte der Neurose-begriffes. *Medizinische Monatsschrift,* 4, 462–4.
Marset, P. (1970). Pinel y el magnetismo animal. *Asclepio,* 22, 219–34.
Marset, P. (1971a). *El punto de partida de la obra psiquiátrica de Pinel.* Valencia (doctoral dissertation).
Marset, P. (1971b). El punto de partida de la obra psiquiátrica de Pinel. Análisis de la producción psiquiátrica de Ph. Pinel anterior al *Traité sur la Manie. Medicina Española,* 65, 390–404.
Marset, P. (1972). Veinte publicaciones psiquiátricas de Pinel olvidadas. Contribución al estudio de los orígenes del *Traité sur la Manie. Episteme,* 6, 163–95.
Marset, P. (1978). La psiquiatría durante la Revolución Francesa: la obra de Philippe Pinel. *Estudios de Historia Social,* 4, 217–87.
McHenry, L. C. (1969). *Garrison's History of Neurology revised and enlarged with a Bibliography of classical, original and Standard Works in Neurology.* Springfield: Thomas.
Meyer, A. & Hierons, R. (1965). On Thomas Willis's Concept of Neurophysiology. *Medical History,* 9, 142–55.
Most, G. F. (1841). *Ueber alte und neue medizinische Lehrsysteme in allgemeine und über J. L. Schönleins neuestes natürliches System der Medizin insbesondere.* Leipzig: Brockhaus.
Mullener, E. R. (1966). Die Rolle der 'passions' in der Psychiatrie des 18. Jahrhunderts. In *Aktuelle Probleme aus der Geschichte der Medizin,* pp. 474–6. Basel & New York: Karger.
Neuburger, M. (1897). *Die historische Entwicklung der experimentellen Gehirn und Rückenmarksphysiologie vor Flourens.* Stuttgart: Enke.
Neuburger, M. (1913). *Johann Christian Reil. Gedenkrede.* Stuttgart: Enke.
Neuburger, M. (1943). British medicine and the Göttingen medical school in the 18th century. *Bulletin of the History of Medicine,* 14, 449–66.
Neuburger, M. (1945). British and German psychiatry in the second half of the eighteenth and the early nineteenth century. *Bulletin of the History of Medicine,* 18, 121–45.
Olmsted, J. (1946). *Charles-Edouard Brown-Séquard, a Nineteenth Century Neurologist and Endocrinologist.* Baltimore: Johns Hopkins Press.
Petzold, I. (1957). Johann Christian Reil, Begründer der modernen Psychotherapie? *Sudhoffs Archiv,* 41, 159–79.
Pfeifer, K. (1968). *Christoph Wilhelm Hufeland, Mensch und Werk.* Halle: Niemeyer.
Rath, G. (1954). Neuralpathologische Anschauungen im 18. Jahrhundert. *Deutsche medizinische Journal,* 5, 125–7.
Rath, G. (1957). Der Kampf zwischen Zellularpathologie und Neuralpathologie im neunzehnten Jahrhundert. *Deutsche medizinische Wochenschrift,* 82, 740–3.

102   *References*

Rather, L. J. (1961). G. E. Stahl's Psychological Physiology. *Bulletin of the History of Medicine*, **25**, 37–49.

Rather, L. J. (1973). G. E. Stahl y F. Hoffmann. In *Historia Universal de la Medicina*, vol. V, ed. P. Laín Entralgo, pp. 326–40. Barcelona: Salvat.

Renvers, R. (1902). Ernst von Leyden als Kliniker. *Deutsche medizinische Wochenschrift*, **28**, 270.

Richardson, B. W. (1890). William Cullen, *Asclepiad*, **7**, 148–77.

Riddell, W. R. (1922). Dr George Cheyne and the 'English Malady'. *Annals of Medical History*, **4**, 304–10.

Riese, W. (1945). History and principles of classification of nervous diseases. *Bulletin of the History of Medicine*, **18**, 465.

Riese, W. (1951). Philippe Pinel (1745–1826). His views on human nature and disease. His medical thought. *Journal of Nervous and Mental Diseases*, **114**, 313–23.

Riese, W. (1965). *La Théorie des Passions à la lumière de la Pensée Médicale du XVIIᵉ Siècle*. Bâle & New York: Karger.

Risse, G. B. (1970). The Brownian system of medicine: its theoretical and practical implications. *Clio Medica*. **5**, 45–51.

Risse, G. B. (1972). Kant, Schelling, and the early search for a philosophical 'Science' of medicine in Germany. *Journal of the History of Medicine*, **27**, 145–58.

Risse, G. B. (1974). 'Doctor William Cullen, Physician, Edinburgh': a consultation practice in the eighteenth century. *Bulletin of the History of Medicine*, **48**, 338–51.

Risse, G. B. (1976). Schelling, 'Naturphilosophie' and John Brown's system of medicine. *Bulletin of the History of Medicine*, **50**, 321–34.

Rosen, G. (1946). The philosophy of ideology and the emergence of modern medicine in France. *Bulletin of the History of Medicine*, **20**, 328–39.

Rosenberg, C. E. (1962). The place of George M. Beard in nineteenth century psychiatry. *Bulletin of the History of Medicine*, **36**, 245–59.

Ruth, T. C. (1946). Charles-Edouard Brown-Séquard (1817–1894). *Yale Journal of Biology and Medicine*, **18**, 227–38.

Schneck, J. M. (1957). Thomas Sydenham and the psychological medicine. *American Journal of Psychiatry*, **113**, 1034–6.

Schneider, D. (1950). *Psychosomatik in der pariser Klinik von Pinel bis Trousseau*. Zürich: Juris (Medizinhistorisches Institut der Universität Zürich).

Schulte, B. P. M. (1959). *Hermanni Boerhaave 'Praelectiones de Morbis nervorum', 1730–1735. Een medisch-historische Studie van Boerhaave's Manuscript over Zenuwziekten*. Leiden: Brill.

Semelaigne, R. (1912). *Aliénistes et Philanthropes. Les Pinel et les Tuke*. Paris: Steinheil.

Semelaigne, R. (1930–32). *Les pionniers de la Psychiatrie française avant et après Pinel*. 2 vols. Paris: Baillière.

Siddall, R. S. (1942). George Cheyne, M.D. eighteenth century clinician and medical author. *Annals of Medical History*, 3rd series, **4**, 95–109.

Skultans, V. (1979). *English Madness. Ideas on Insanity, 1580–1890*. London: Routledge & Kegan Paul.

Stapples, F. (1897). William Cullen. *New York Medical Journal*, **66**, 689–91.

Steiner, A. (1954). *Das nervöse Zeitalter. Der Begriff der Nervosität bei Laien und Aerzten in Deutschland und Oesterreich um 1910*. Zürich: Juris (Medizinhistorisches Institut der Universität Zürich).

Temkin, O. (1957). A critique of medical historiography. In *On the Utility of Medical History*, ed. I. Galdston, pp. 21–34. New York: International Universities Press.

Temkin, O. (1971). *The Falling Sickness. A History of Epilepsy from the Greeks to the Beginnings of Modern Neurology*. 2nd edn. Baltimore: The Johns Hopkins Press.

Thomson, J., Thomson, W. & Craigie, D. (1832). *An Account of the Life, Lectures and Writings of William Cullen*. 2 vols. Edinburgh: Blackwood.

Turban, K. L. (1950). *Georg Ernst Stahl als Vorläufer der modernen Psychosomatik*. München (doctoral dissertation).

Veith, I. (1956). On hysterical and hypochondriacal affections. *Bulletin of the History of Medicine*, **30**, 233–40.

Veith, I. (1960). Philippe Pinel and the moral treatment of insanity. *Modern Medicine*, **28**, 212–26.

Veith, I. (1965). *Hysteria. The History of a Disease*. Chicago: Chicago University Press.

Wettley, A. (1959). Hysterie, ärztliche Einbildung oder Wirklichkeit? *Münchener medizinische Wochenschrift*, **101**, 193–6.

Woods, E. A. & Carlson, E. T. (1961). The psychiatry of Philippe Pinel. *Bulletin of the History of Medicine*, **25**, 37–42.

Index

105

106

Index